NURSING :

Beyond Tradition and Conflict

Editors

Moya Jolley

MA (Ed), BSc (Econ), DipEd (Lond), RGN,
RNT, DipN (Lond)

and

Gosia Brykczynska

BSc, BA, RGN, RSCN, DipPH, Cert Ed,
OnCert, RNT

Foreword by
Alison Kitson

⋈ Mosby

London Baltimore Bogotá Boston Buenos Aires Caracas Carlsbad, CA Chicago Madrid Mexico City Milan Naples, FL
New York Philadelphia St. Louis Sydney Tokyo Toronto Wiesbaden

Project Manager:	Roddy Craig
Publisher:	Griselda Campbell
Editorial Consultant:	Nancy Loffler
Production:	Joe Lynch
Index:	Lisa Weinkove
Design:	Judith Gauge
Cover Design:	Lara Last

Published in 1995 by Mosby, an imprint of Times Mirror International Publishers Limited

Printed by J W Arrowsmiths Ltd

ISBN 0 7234 19523

For full details of all Times Mirror International Publishers Limited titles, please write to Times Mirror International Publishers Limited, Lynton House, 7–12 Tavistock Square, London WC1H 9LB, UK.

A CIP catalogue record for this book is available from the British Library.

CONTENTS

THE EDITORS

Moya Jolley MA (Ed), BSc (Econ),
DipEd (Lond), RGN, RNT, DipN (Lond)
Formerly lecturer in Sociology
Institute of Advanced Nursing Education
Royal College of Nursing
London

Gosia Brykczynska BSc, BA, RGN, RSCN,
DipPH, Cert Ed, OnCert, RNT
Lecturer in Ethics and Philosophy
Institute of Advanced Nursing Education
Royal College of Nursing
London

CONTRIBUTORS

Alan Myles MA (Ed), DipEd, RGN, RNT
Vice Principal
Institute of Advanced Nursing Education
Royal College of Nursing, London

Diane Marks-Maran BSc RGN DipN (Lond) RNT
Head of Resource-Based Learning
School of Health and Science
Thames Valley University

Robert Garbett RGN, BN (Hons)
Project Worker/Team Leader
7E Development Unit
Oxford Radcliffe NHS Trust

Ann Keen RN DN PGCEA
General Secretary
Community and District Nurses Association

Christine Hancock BSc (Econ) RGN
General Secretary
Royal College of Nursing. London

FOREWORD

It is beginning to be accepted and understood that we live in a complex and rapidly changing world. If we believe the post-modernists then we are faced with making sense of a multiplicity of ideas, attitudes, behaviours and actions, all acceptable within limits, all permissible within cultural and personal acceptability.

Slipping into such relativism, is, on the surface, acceptable even to be desired; yet the consequences are quite profound. It is the clear message of this book that there may be certain universal truths or positions which need to be taken in order to move nursing onwards. The discussion on the nature of knowledge is important for this reason. Does knowledge come from within or do we become wiser people by acquiring facts? If the cultivation of personal wisdom is a pre-requisite for establishing and sustaining a profession known for its compassion, skill and caring ability, then do we have sufficient members willing to engage in this? To what extent do nurses really want to be wise, heroic, or martyrs? And are there a set of universal values which are immutable despite the push towards relativism?

These questions are raised in the opening chapter of the book and serve as a beacon to guide the reader through the following pages. From the intellectual discussions of how models and theories can be used to improve practice we are brought to think about the impact of educational reforms, politics and future health needs on the practice of nursing.

Rightly no answers are given; many questions are asked and the reader is challenged to reflect upon his or her own understanding and commitment to making nursing better. To summarise what the authors communicated to my understanding of nursing is to echo Schweitzer, where he said that in order to subcribe to a notion of progress and civilisation it is necessary to manifest hope and think optimistically.

The style of this book is erudite, witty, poignant and direct. It challenges the reader to think about the basic values of compassion, courage and caring. It is an optimistic book, perhaps because it seeks to remind each one of us that the destiny of the nursing profession is not in the hands of outsiders or politicians but in the hands of each individual who calls him- or herself a nurse, knowing what that means and having the courage to be it.

Dr Alison Kitson
Director
National Institute for Nursing
Centre for Practice Development and Research
Oxford
1995

PREFACE

Ever since Florence Nightingale founded the modern nursing profession, standards of care, initially improved in comparison with the situation prior to 1860, have been continually vulnerable to a multiplicity of forces from both within and without the occupation.

As is well recognised, care is influenced by, among other things, economic, political, and social forces externally; and professional, bureaucratic, manpower and attitudinal factors internally. That these tensions have gathered momentum over the past decade appears to be self evident. That they may continue to do so is a serious cause for concern.

This book seeks to explore some of the issues involved, to delineate areas of conflict and tension – both internally and externally – and to tentatively explore possible ways forward.

The opening chapter addresses current nursing practices utilizing philosophical and ethical perspectives. It seeks to analyse the extent to which nurses are providing care that can be seen to be a compromise version of their original caring ideals. It looks at the nature of wisdom and its relationship to caring. Chapter 3 explores the problems related to the use and misuse of nursing models. The theme of caring is further expanded in the following chapter which examines the theory/practice gap, and its implications for standards of care. The reform process in modern nursing education, the problems associated with ongoing curriculum renewal, and the establishment of Project 2000 courses are examined in Chapter 2, whilst the substance of Chapter 5 deals with internal professional development, relationships, images, and stereotypes old and new. Chapter 6 explores some recent political issues affecting health care workers, while the closing chapter seeks to address possible future developments and ways forward in a rapidly changing profession.

Each chapter is capable of standing alone, whilst also contributing to the overall analysis of some of the acute problems confronting the nursing profession as it attempts to fulfil its major function of caring.

Moya Jolley
Gosia Brykczynska
London
1995

ACKNOWLEDGMENTS

The editors would like to extend their grateful thanks to all the contributors to this book. Their interest, enthusiasm, and willingness to give of their time and expertise is what makes the production of books such as this possible. Thanks also go to Dr Alison Kitson for writing the foreword; also to Mrs Jean Smith and Mrs Elizabeth Hillman for typing various chapters and Miss Maria Bninska for help in preparation of the manuscript. We wish also to extend our grateful thanks, once again, to Miss Helen Thomas, Assistant Librarian in the Library of Nursing at the Royal College of Nursing for her continued help in the meticulous checking and preparation of references.

Lastly our thanks go to Mrs Nancy Loffler, Editorial Consultant – Mosby, for her help and support during the preparation of this book.

1.

REFLECTIVE PRACTICE: AN ANALYSIS OF NURSING WISDOM

Nurses are currently being urged by their leaders to be 'reflective practitioners'. What is not clear, however, is to what extent nurses are to 'reflect', and on what subjects are they urged to meditate so earnestly (Shön, 1983). In a world and politico-economic climate where 'standing and staring' is considered a waste of time and equated with social vice, it is worth considering what exactly nurses' leaders had in mind when they made the call for more reflection in practice.

Taking time out to reflect on our actions appears a laudable undertaking until we consider that reflection, by definition, can be a thoroughly passive process whereby a substance or mirror or other polished surface reflects or throws back, so to speak, light or heat, an image even, that has been projected onto it, or that has fallen upon it. As the *Shorter Oxford English Dictionary* (1973) states, reflection is the 'action of a mirror or other polished surface in exhibiting or reproducing the image of an object . . . the action of bending, turning or folding back' (all no doubt referring to the use of the word in the context of physics and optics, but not very helpful in the immediate instance, in the context of professional practice). One of the secondary definitions of the word, however, refers to 'the action of turning (back) or fixing the thoughts on some subject; meditation, deep or serious consideration . . . recollection or rememberance of a thing'.

In a philosophical context, reflection can be considered 'the mode, operation or faculty by which the mind has knowledge of itself and its operations, or by which it deals with the ideas received from sensation and perception . . . a thought or idea occurring to, or occupying the mind . . . a thought expressed in words' (*Shorter Oxford English Dictionary*, 1973).

Thus the word 'reflection' conveys the notion of optically, that is, physically, reproducing an image or a perception of reality, and also, by extension, its meaning has broadened to include the notion of 'reflecting' back an idea, or a cognitive perception, such as remembrance or even the very act of thinking and meditating itself. Thus reflection in the second sense, of reflecting an idea or meditating (by being made aware of) or 'turning back' some cover of practice to discover what lies beneath is closer to our nursing use of the word.

The notion of reflection as pertaining to the 'throwing back', or 'reflection' of an idea, is an attractive one; it has, however, some rather obvious inherent flaws, namely, that the ideas reflected back, made clearer, or simply held up for examination must firstly be seen to come from somewhere concrete (one can only reflect what actually is seen to exist). Secondly, how would the passive reflector (in this case the nurse) achieve reflective qualities – as presumably not all substances (beings) are equally reflective. Finally, we can only recognize reflection in optics and physics because of our visual and tactile senses (we can, for example, sense the reflection of sound or heat), but how do we know that we have 'reflected' a thought, notion or idea, or that we have even meditated upon something? What are the senses used (if any) that would indicate to ourselves and others that a thought, idea, notion or whatever has been 'reflected', that is, 'turned back', meditated upon and projected 'outward' for examination?

These are not pointless speculations; they are in fact the essence of philosophical argumentation, and the very basis of epistemology, which has been defined as 'the philosophical theory of knowledge, which seeks to define it, distinguish its principle varieties, identify its sources, and establish its limits' (Bullock and Stallybrass, 1977). How we know something, and how we know that we know, and whether or not something constitutes knowledge or truth are all the subject matter of epistemology and of vital relevance to our discussion. The reflection that we are urged to undertake, the 'serious consideration' of practice, can only be sensibly undertaken if we understand what it is that that particular reflection involves; that we can recognize it when we see it, and that we are prepared to face its implications when it is projected for us to view. The analogy is, however, a precarious one, for how often do we really need to thoroughly understand a word to be able to use it correctly? The problem lies in our professional capacity to be seen to control the concept, rather than have the meanings of the concept dictate to us how we are to proceed. Any other position enslaves us instead of promoting our intellectual freedom – thus we tend to become enslaved by ideas that we do not really understand. In nursing, for example, the idealization of research has led many nurses to think that they personally should conduct nursing research. They have become slaves to the research idea. An elaboration of the concept 'reflection' is therefore useful, so that it is clear to all concerned what is meant by the term.

I will attempt to demonstrate that professional 'reflection' is not possible without personal wisdom, that wisdom is far more than mere knowledge, and that the wisdom referred to by philosophers, theologians and writers is the very essence of that 'reflection' that is urged upon us by our professional leaders, even if this is not what they originally had in mind in issuing that particular directive.

The first task at hand, therefore, is to analyse the concept of wisdom. What do we mean when we talk about someone being wise? What is this thing called wisdom?

Aristotle saw wisdom as one of five intellectual virtues. Lloyd (1968) translates these virtues as art, scientific knowledge, rational intuition, practical intelligence and wisdom. Furthermore, wisdom, according to Aristotle, was seen as a combination of 'the faculty whereby we get knowledge of the first principles or starting points from which such demonstrations begin', and 'scientific knowledge', where these 'related to the highest and most valuble objects'. This type of 'wisdom' has also been variously translated as 'intelligence' or 'intellectual excellence' and indeed Chapters 1 and 2 of Book Six of Aristotle's *Nichomachean Ethics* analyses intellectual excellence, i.e. 'kinds of intellectual excellences and their objects'. However, it is not until Chapters 5, 6 and 7 that we start to recognize definitions of wisdom as we would use the word today. This should not surprise us, as of all the virtues described by Aristotle, wisdom was and is one of the most hard to grasp intellectually. Indeed it is a virtue not all of us are keen to be identified with. It is as if it were possible to be 'too wise', or as if whatever cluster of psychological and social attributes follow wisdom these were seen as not altogether positive. Certainly, we hear of nurses who prefer to be 'doers' rather than 'thinkers', equating 'thinking activities' with a kind of intellectual irresponsibility corresponding to an extravagant, luxurious, 'ivory-tower' life-style. 'Nice nurses are simply not like that', they would claim.

Aristotle, however, saw wisdom as consisting of aspects of practicality (especially in referring to practical wisdom), intelligence, abstractness, theoretical conciseness, shrewdness and perception (when wisdom is combined with politics and rationality, as would be seen in 'excellence in deliberation'). Additional to these ideas come notions of understanding (good sense) and moral virtue. Thus, Aristotle saw wisdom as encompassing notions of enactment, requiring at least a minimal level of intelligence or intellectual ability, an approach to reasoning that was primarily abstract in nature, logical and systematic, necessitating a practical knowledge to be fruitful, based on a level of sensibility that would order ideas and prioritize them, and finally crowned with a perception of morality that would be seen as an integral virtue of the 'wise' person. Aristotle claims 'that it is impossible to be good in the full sense of the word without practical wisdom or to be a man of practical wisdom without moral excellence or virtue'. Indeed, Aristotle considered wisdom to be the Principle Virtue that binds together all other virtues, claiming that as soon as man 'possesses this single virtue of practical wisdom, he will also possess all the rest' (Aristotle, 1962, Book 6, Chapter 13, 1145a).

So far it would be difficult to argue that a contemporary nurse should be anything else but an exemplar of Aristotelian wisdom. Wisdom, to the Greeks of Aristotle's time, consisted in an ability to successfully deliberate about important issues, about 'what sort of thing contributes to the good life in general' (Aristotle, 1962, Book 6, Chapter 5). Such ethical deliberations are vital to the well-being of a modern nurse.

Men with 'practical wisdom', according to Aristotle, have the 'capacity of seeing what is good for themselves and for mankind, and these are, we believe, the qualities of men capable of managing households and states' (Aristotle, 1962, Book 6, Chapter 5). If we consider the qualities needed for a good practising nurse, surely this 'practical wisdom' of which Aristotle speaks is one of the essential virtues we would cast aside at our peril. There is an element of caution in Aristotle's consideration of practical wisdom, however, for he does not see it as a quality that can be entirely learnt or acquired (or that we could train ourselves to acquire): 'it is not merely a rational characteristic or trained ability. An indication (that is something more may be seen) is the fact that a trained ability of that kind can be forgotten, whereas practical wisdom cannot' (Aristotle: 1962, Book 6, Chapter 5).

Aristotle saw the role of intelligence as necessary to 'apprehend' fundamental principles of science, scientific knowledge and theoretical wisdom, much as the profession of nursing would require a minimal level of intelligence in its practitioners to ensure adequate interpretation of nursing data, facts and phenomena. There are countless examples of nursing auxillaries casually recording ominous information on patients' health status notes because they lacked sufficient depth of understanding to correctly interpret the data. Needless to say, examples can be cited of untrained workers demonstrating more intelligence than educated professionals, but that does not alter the fundamental observation, as noted by Aristotle, that essential intelligence is not something that, once socio-culturally and genetically acquired, can be forgotten. It certainly can be encouraged to flourish and develop, but as a quality necessary for wisdom, it cannot be a transitory, whimsical, or purely trained phenomenon.

Aristotle differentiates theoretical wisdom from practical wisdom. He considers theoretical wisdom as general and abstract, far from relevance to everyday deliberations over correct conduct or even interpretations of the everyday phenomena that characterize practical wisdom. Thus he says, 'theoretical wisdom must comprise both intelligence and scientific knowledge. It is science in its consummation, as it were, the science of the things that are valued most highly' (Aristotle, 1962, Book 6, Chapter 7). He therefore considers it quite possible to have theoretical wisdom, but not practical wisdom, giving the example of Anaxagoras and Thales who 'do not know what is advantageous to them . . . they know extraordinary, wonderful, difficult, and superhuman things, but call their knowledge useless because the good they are seeking is not human . . . Practical wisdom, on the other hand, is concerned with human affairs and with matters about which deliberation is possible' (Aristotle, 1962, Book 6, Chapter 7). Practical wisdom encompasses major universal concerns, and uses the skills of deliberation. It is far more focused on human concerns and entirely dependent on humane morally good interpretations as achieved through contemplation of life and having a reservoir of positive experience. Theoretical wisdom, however, can be achievable at a very early age and does not necessarily concern itself with 'ultimate particulars' but rather scientific and philosophical principles. Finally, Aristotle points out the truism noted by many arm-chair psychologists even today, that 'a young man has no experience, for experience is the product of a long time. In fact, one might also raise the question why it is that a boy may become a mathematician but not a philosopher or a natural scientist. The answer may be that the objects of mathematics are the result of abstraction, whereas the fundamental principles of philosophy and natural science come from experience' (Aristotle, 1962, Book 6, Chapter 8).

If we saw nursing as a perfect marriage of philosophy and natural science it might shed some light on the understanding that wisdom in such a context would take quite a while to develop and that the scientific facts and knowledge relevant to the art of nursing can be learnt fairly easily, but they would not, without specific additional catalytic input, become transformed into wisdom, not even practical nursing wisdom. Wisdom as perceived by Aristotle is a supreme virtue because it represents an entire personal approach and life-style of the 'wise person'. Practical wisdom is not therefore a commodity, as knowledge may be, it is an internalized virtue that speaks to a level of moral development rather than scholastic achievements that can be reached in encyclopedic knowledge.

At this point someone may well say that there is surely more than one definition of wisdom, and, moreover, that the concept of wisdom has changed over the centuries. An analysis will therefore be presented of various scholars' and sages' understanding of wisdom, and its relationship with knowledge and life-style.

Naturally, concepts of wisdom are not confined to the writings of ancient Greek philosophers. The nature of the truly wise person, the essence of wisdom and the nature of the acquisition of knowledge has interested scholars unrelentingly for thousands of years. Each age and period in man's history corresponds to new attempts to redefine the essence of knowledge and the nature of wisdom, and we are offered ever anew contemporary models of the wise person. Interestingly it is not only men, but also women philosophers who have had much to say on the subject of wisdom, the acquisition of knowledge and active reflection. Counter-balancing Francis Bacon's brilliant exposé, written in the seventeeth century, on the studiousness required of the wise person – 'To spend too much time on studies is sloth; to use them too much for ornament is affectation; to make judgement wholly by their rules is the humour of a scholar' (Bacon, 1973, p.150) – are the measured writings of female scholars, especially medieval female scholars. It also needs to be said, if only in passing, that the wise person is not necessarily a 'studious' person, i.e. an individual who 'knows' many facts and studies them. Acquisition of wisdom is not synonymous with acquisition of 'knowledge' or what Aristotle would call theoretical wisdom, and which Bacon referred to as the 'false point of wisdom', or 'cunning' (Bacon, 1973 p.150). 'We take cunning for a sinister or crooked wisdom. And certainly there is a great difference between a cunning man and a wise man, not only in point of honesty, but in point of ability' (Bacon, 1973 p.68). Bacon rightly fits scholarship into perspective as regards wisdom, commenting that 'crafty men condemn studies; simple men admire them; and wise men use them, for they teach not their own use but that there is a wisdom without them and above them, won by observation' (Bacon,1973 p.150). Thus, the wisdom we refer to is the total disposition of the individual, a result of intellectual ability and virtuous reflection – a state of being much closer to Aristotle's practical wisdom than any other concept.

Women in the past have had to strive hard to prove their intellectual ability, and often (even if it was fostered in childhood), it was socially discouraged in the mature woman. Some women, however, managed to cultivate intellectual abilities in spite of social norms antagonistic towards them. The practical wisdom developed by these women became the fruit of true learning and (at least initially) uniquely female insights, reflections and emphasis. The reflection and thinking brought about by women to illuminate scholarship (which was largely male dominated) were tempered by virtues that Aristotle himself would have recognized, and which contributed to the growth and progress of civilization in medieval Europe.

As the excellent series *A History of Women Philosophers* demonstrates, female philosophers, thinkers and writers, from ancient Greece to contemporary times, have profoundly influenced the worlds in which they have lived, and manifested a collective wisdom equal to, and often different from, the accepted male scholastic wisdom of their times (Waithe, 1989).

If we accept that there is no genetic reason why a woman should display intellectual abilities inferior to a man's, barring socio-cultural conditionings, the qualitative differences in wisdom, if they are present at all, manifested by women philosophers, theologians, writers and mystics are most probably due to the nature of a woman's reflection and experience. Characteristic of female philosophers, especially the medieval mystics, was their emphasis on the value of the virtues of charity and love in promoting wisdom. This was strikingly different from the writings of their contemporary male peers, such as Duns Scotus or Aquinas, brilliant and wise men who were much less concerned with aspects of the 'affective domain' (Waithe, 1989).

Women saw the need to temper their intellectual abilities with a sense of all-embracing charity and love, often it would seem at the expense of their own intellectual prowess. Thus, Marie le Jars de Gournay, the French essayist and friend of Montaigne, excused women's subordinate place in the world by saying satirically 'that what constitutes [a woman's] only happiness and [her] only sovereign virtue is to be ignorant, to be foolish, and to serve' (Zedler, 1989, p.301). In reality, some women could be seen as wise counsellors as much as men, respected for their unique insights and truly 'female' wisdom. Women like Hildegard of Bingen, Mechtild of Magdeburg and Hadewych of Antwerp represent the best of medieval female ecclesiastical scholarship and are also examplary of whole schools of learning (Waithe, 1989), much consulted by their male colleagues. Indeed, women were sometimes as learned or even more learned than their male counterparts, as the example of Heloise studying in Paris attests to, but not all famous, witty and learned medieval women could be considered wise. Wise women, that is, women possessing the quality of practical wisdom as well as intellectual powers, were usually also virtuous in the Aristotelian sense, and often possessed mystical qualities. Thus, Mother Julian of Norwich, the English medieval mystic, was a woman who has been considered by many over the centuries to be endowed with 'practical wisdom' (Evasdaughter, 1989).

Julian herself, commenting on the source of her wisdom, states that it was a divine gift, an attribute that she was grateful for, but could not totally control, except by the practice of virtue. She notes that it is God who 'of his goodness he opens the eye of our understanding so that we can see; sometimes it is less, sometimes more, according to our God-given ability to receive it' (Upjohn, 1992, Chapter 25). Wise women such as Catherine of Siena, Brigitta of Sweden and many German abbesses were confidants and counsellors of noblemen, prelates, even Emperors and Popes. Taking the counsel of wise people, male or female, was then as now a common practice. As Bacon (1973) noted, 'The wisest princes need not think it any diminution to their greatness, or derogation to their sufficiency, to rely upon counsel. God himself is not without, but hath made it one of the great names of his blessed Son: The Counsellor . . .' (p.62).

It is therefore of interest that so many of the great, wise women of the middle-ages saw the concepts of love and knowledge that they most often had in mind in terms of the divine. Contemporary men, though much indebted to the female mystics and philosophers, spoke a different language. They played a different tune, so to speak. As Evasdaughter (1989) observes about Julian of Norwich's *Showings*, 'she held that knowledge of God results in love, that knowledge is necessary to love God, that knowledge is characteristic of divine love and that knowledge is among the gifts God's love gives us' (p.217). Considerably later, in the sixteenth century, Thomas More's daughter, Margaret Roper, distinguished herself by her pursuance of scholastic excellence, but she succeeded in tempering it with a courageous love of her father and her faith that has rarely been witnessed in the course of history (Waithe, 1989). Indeed she manifested a particular form of wisdom, one that let a courageous love shape her intellectual abilities and senses. Perhaps it was a wisdom akin to the ancient wisdom displayed by Antigone, or the belated, medieval scholastic wisdom of hindsight of Heloise, or the spiritual home-spun wisdom of Julian of Norwich. Certainly Julian, compared to the others, would hardly have been considered to have outstanding intellectual ability or even courage, but she was considered nonetheless to be wise and knowledgeable about things that mattered, especially the soul. Manifestations of wisdom therefore vary, demonstrating a creativity of approach that is boundless and controlled only by the limitations of the human spirit. Female wisdom, additionally, is tinged with overt counsel regarding love of the other and charity. It is characteristically concerned with promoting love, encouraging charity and interpersonal understanding. It is often based on a sense of altruism – a womanly concern with 'reaching out'. Thus Catherine of Siena writes about a 'bridge of love', and Teresa of Avila about rooms in a 'divine mansion' (very female orientated pictures, full of homely imagery). All these evaluations of the nature of wisdom demonstrated by medieval women could be successfully transferred to a description of optimal modern nursing characteristics. Certainly there is an affinity between the 'wisdom' manifested by these women and the wisdom required for nursing practices today.

Julian of Norwich in Chapter 5 of her *Showings* tells us about 'a little thing, the size of a hazelnut in the palm of my hand' (Upjohn, 1992, p.4) which signifies all of created matter. If all of created matter is so insignificant as this hazelnut compared to the wonder and glory of God, Julian adds, how can anything less than God satisfy us? This literal, home-spun (infused) spiritual wisdom, which is akin to the mystical insights re-iterated countless times by many theologians and philosophers the world over and which is independent of cultural variables, is representative of a female spiritual creativity that is gentle and at the same time powerful. To recognize one's insignificance in the face of the universe, and the insignificance of this realization in face of the Might and Love of God, is as much an imagery of power as it is of gentleness.

Modern considerations of wisdom, however, are as much touched by secular humanism as they are by the call for moral integrity. The language of ethics has taken the place of theology, and modern science is now the subject matter of revelation and metaphysics. Modern wisdom is necessarily centred on the concerns of modern man. However, that wisdom manifested by wise people is, as always, as much 'other-regarding' as was the wisdom of the ancient Greeks or medieval female mystics. Each age re-interprets for itself the meaning of wisdom, but true wisdom, devoid of cultural trappings, never loses its 'other-regarding' and outward-looking qualities. A knowledgeable, but conceited and self-centred person who is wrapped up in the concerns of minutiae may be a useful person to society in a particular instance, but would not be deemed to possess 'practical wisdom'.

Wisdom is devoid of the need for specific details that an abundance of knowledge presupposes. However, there is a modern intellectual heresy, sometimes seen even in nursing circles, that claims that an abundance of knowledge, especially in the form of 'facts', leads necessarily to excellence of reasoning and therefore excellence of practice knowledge.

The wise person can often make sense of a whole phenomena by giving startling creative examples, and it is this startling creativity that betrays the depths of their wisdom. The teachings of Indian gurus, Chinese Buddhist monks and the Desert Fathers of the fourth century AD all demonstrate this ability. Their insights are based on personal growth, not on frantically collected facts and figures.

Wisdom is also characteristically and, by definition, gentle and forgiving. Knowledge has no such ethical obligations or, indeed, such leeway in its formal or informal structures.

The secular humanism that permeates modern notions of wisdom is represented at its best in the value of contemporary man as characterized by Iris Murdoch: 'Human beings are valuable, not because they are created by God or because they are rational beings or good citizens, but because they are human beings' (*Metaphysics as a Guide to Morals* 1992, p.365). This is a very modern image of the value of man, infused with modern moral insights.

Modern philosophers and historians of science, such as Michel Polanyi (1962), Thomas Kuhn (1962) and Karl Popper (1972), have tried to define and delineate the scope and limitations of the idea of contemporary scientific knowledge and science. Knowledge, as noted by Aristotle, is an integral aspect of wisdom, and therefore its constraints will always be of interest to the wise person. For contemporary man, knowledge will be seen as internalized scientific knowledge and hopefully, in time, will become 'knowledge by acquaintance' (Russell, 1967). Polanyi, however, is not at all sure where this scientific knowledge starts and where it may finish, how it is transmitted and, even more significantly, how it is revised in the light of new, contradictory material. If knowledge were but a collection of objectively known facts, codification of them and the ensuing science would result in the formation of rigorous taxonomies. This task might be scholastically possible (though not without its own internal classificatory hazards), as is witnessed by the present goal of The Human Genome Project. All of the human genes found on Watson and Crick's DNA double helix, which constitutes the living matter of human life, are to be isolated, identified and classified. This is a laborious undertaking, and one carried out by elaborate computers, not wise men (or women). It would appear to be true, therefore, as Polanyi (1962) notes, that 'science is operated by the skill of the scientist and it is through the exercise of his skill that he shapes his scientific knowledge' (p.49). By leaving computers (albeit programmed by scientists) to do much of the 'discovering', the human scientists becomes impoverished and his wisdom curtailed. Again, it is Polanyi (1962) who warns that 'personal knowledge in science is not made but discovered, and as such it claims to establish contact with reality beyond the clues on which it relies' (p.64). Can computerized, in effect second-hand, knowledge, ever be transformed into personal knowledge as envisaged by Polanyi or even Russell (1967), a hundred years ago? For Polanyi (1962), science is an all-engrossing passion, much as studying classical texts was for the monastic scholars of previous generations: 'it commits us, passionately and far beyond our comprehension, to a vision of reality. Of this responsibility we cannot divest ourselves by setting up objective criteria of verifiability or falsifiability or testability or what you will. For we live in it as in the garment of our own skin' (p.64). For Polanyi, scientists are responsible for their science (and knowledge) precisely because they themselves embody scientific knowledge. It is personal responsibility and identification with scientific knowledge that pushes Polanyi's description of knowledge into the realm of moral philosophy and morality; it betrays the presence of wisdom. Thus the statement now joins the language of ethics rather than that of empiricism and traditionally understood modern science. It brings Polanyi's work into the realm of moral philosophy, which has a language and vocabulary also shared by those who possess wisdom. The wise person sees the whole, and always strives to find unity, ever endeavouring to bring about creativity. This is nothing more than an 'awareness of particulars which compromise a whole' (Polanyi, 1962, p.65).

Karl Popper, the philosopher of science who so profoundly influenced contemporary notions of knowledge, especially scientific knowledge, claims to have replaced the tradition of the idea of knowledge that went back to the time of Aristotle by an 'objective theory of essentially conjectural knowledge' (Popper, 1972, Preface). According to Popper (1972), subjectivist commonsense knowledge has hindered the progress of science. He states that he disagrees with almost all scientific theoreticians, except Charles Darwin and Albert Einstein (two giants of modern science who were themselves essentially theoreticians, rather than activists), over a general definition of a theory of knowledge and knowledge generation. He asserts 'that the growth of knowledge proceeds from old problems to new problems, by means of conjectures and refutations' (p.258). He states that although we may be born or start off with a form of hypothetical knowledge, it is itself the core of our first problem, 'and ensuing growth of our knowledge may therefore be described as consisting throughout of corrections and modifications of previous knowledge' (p.259). This concept of the growth of knowledge in the scientific world echoes in some interesting ways the explanations given by mystics as to how their knowledge is increased and confirmed. Only occasionally are bursts of insights allowed and even then these soon become incorporated into a vision of the whole. The manifestation of 'practical wisdom' is not so much dependent on revelationary momentary insights, which sometimes occur in the world of science, as on reflection and the processing of internalized experiences. Wisdom, as noted by Aristotle, takes time to develop.

It is noteworthy, therefore, that for Popper (1974), man appears more likely to die for ideas and to defend what he believes in (that is, has personal knowledge of), rather than reason (that is, rationality). Hence he states: 'Man, we may say, appears to be not so much a rational animal as an ideological animal' (p.1149). Ideas are the building blocks of knowledge, but considered ideas become the foundation of personal knowledge – they contribute to wisdom. The question remains, however, whether this passion for ideas manifested by the ordinary man is conducive to fostering true wisdom, or is the 'evolutionary approach' inherent in Popper's theory of promotion of scientific knowledge closer to reality? Certainly, it is clear that it is not the acquisition or promotion of knowledge alone or even virtue and its inherent merits that constitutes true wisdom. Wisdom, even for the contemporary, 'science-drunk' person is more than 'mere knowledge'. This is an observation that nurses could well professionally reflect on. The pursuit of knowledge must also be accompanied by personal reflection and scholastic proportioning of values.

Michel Polanyi and Harry Prosch (1975) noted that it is the mechanical reductionism and scientific obscurantism that explains 'the corruption of the conception of man' (p.25), the latter being one of the main concerns of the wise person. They also accuse modern science of reducing man 'either to an insentient automaton or to a bundle of appetites' (p.25). Neither of these results of modern scholarship seem to reflect the holism necessary for a humanistic approach to man. It is interesting to ponder how they would view 'New Age scientists' on the one hand and contemporary gene-hunting geneticists on the other. It is also interesting that this total extremism in approaches appears to hinder knowledge and scientific progress, which Polanyi and Prosch (1975) considered as denying scientists the possibility of assuming personal responsibility for their science, knowledge and perceptions of man. Such yearnings for an ethical, holistic approach to the understanding and promotion of scientific knowledge, written over twenty years ago, still needs to be addressed today. It is the kernal of concerns for the modern, secular, humanistic, and learned fraternity of committed scholars, some of whom are undeniably wise, and some of whom are also nurses.

The question one could well address now is: what is the association between these concepts of knowledge and 'practical wisdom' and the profession of nursing as it is practised today? Knowledge, as contemporary philosophers consider it, is 'that of which one can speak in a discursive practice, and which is specified by the fact: the domain constituted by the different objects that will or will not acquire a scientific status . . . Knowledge is also the space in which the subject may take up a position and speak of the objects with which he deals in his discourse . . . lastly knowledge is defined by the possibilities of use and appropriation offered by discourse' (Foucault, 1972 p.183). Knowledge, as understood by Foucault in this passage, involves the intelligent perception of facts, absorption of interrelated data and a debate concerning the conclusions. Knowledge for him is not a collection of isolated facts, unconnected to a broader or wider sense of reality. Certainly, a raw unprocessed taxonomy (even of human genes), as we have seen, would not qualify as knowledge for him; the taxonomy would have to fit into a discourse on human anatomy and physiology, specifically genetics, in order to be qualified as medical scientific knowledge. It is of note, therefore, that he categorically states that there is 'no knowledge without a particular discursive practice; and any discursive practice may be defined by the knowledge that it forms' (Foucault, 1972 p.183). In relation to nursing knowledge and nursing practice, some nurse-theoreticians claim that there is not yet an extant body of knowledge related to nursing that could be regarded as representative of the discipline, while others disagree. Certainly, a philosopher of science such as Foucault would not have too much difficulty given his definitions of scientific knowledge in defining nursing knowledge where there is a 'particular discursive practice . . . defined by the knowledge that it forms' (Foucault, 1972 p.183).

Robert Neville, in a philosophic monograph on 'aspects of spiritual development', explains, as a philosopher, his attempts to 'provide a way of seeing things in context and in connection with other things, which is not available from the standpoint of the enterprise under investigation' (Neville, 1978). He defines in the work the knowledge necessary for 'the sage' and it is the sage, that is, 'the wise person', that is of prime importance to us (Neville, 1978 p. 47). For him, knowledge is a way of possessing something, of taking it in: 'The knower appropriates the object known . . . We can know particular objects through time and we can have theoretical knowledge of types of objects and how they would be at any time' (Neville, 1978 p.47). Such definitions of knowledge, as if it were a collection of objects to be identified (metaphorically, the ingestion of facts – of their possession), is not new. To the nurse such definitions of knowledge may give rise to momentary considerations, such as whether or not the contemporary discipline of nursing is based on 'particular discursive practices', e.g. the knowledge concerning pain control in palliative care. It is of interest to what extent a nurse's knowledge of particular facts, which build up a practical perspective from which she can predict certain other facts, e.g. lack of holistic intervention for the terminally ill patient who is in uncontrolled pain, is likely to be effective. The ability to knowledgeably predict a course of events can only be based on the acceptance of certain premises, which themselves form a basis of knowledge. I would argue that nursing has a body of knowledge, if somewhat limited, but that which is more significant is the knowledge base of its individual practitioners, and also their level of personal self-knowledge. It is predominantly personal, i.e. total life knowledge, levels of self-knowledge that ultimately determine levels of sagacity, that is, of practical wisdom, rather than levels of intensity of solely 'professional knowledge', which would equate more to Aristotle's theoretical wisdom.

Neville (1978) says of self-knowledge that it should lead to a true self-image, that is, an honest appraisal of one's desires, patterned ideals, actual strivings and goals. He states that it is both painful and difficult to hold up the mirror of truth; that we often do not know what it is we are looking at and delude ourselves as to the nature of reality, like socratic cavemen observing hidden shadows (Plato, 1974). Yet, he adds, 'the interest of self-knowledge is not the technical one of satisfying the desires, but the cognitive one of discovering who one is . . . what one really believes and what one really wants are connected with what one really wills' (Neville, 1978 p.52). It is knowing what we really want that shapes who we really are. Philosophers have long debated the problems of free will and pre-determinism and modern sociologists have only added to the complexities of the argument, but the philosopher would always add, that at a minimum, knowledge of where one wants to be and knowledge of what one wants (i.e. wishes and desires, in philosophical terms, wills), even given socio-cultural conditionings and limitations, must be better than unreflective drifting, wherever life's vagaries will take us. It is the understanding of self that is necessary in order to be considered wise. If a profession were striving for wisdom as opposed to 'mere knowledge', it too would need to undertake a similar form of self-appraisal.

It is interesting that nursing as a profession has attempted an exercise of self-appraisal, which upon occasion has been brutal and self-condemning (*see* Jolley, 1989), whereas according to many psychologists and philosophers of human nature, self-knowledge should lead to humility not self-condemnation. Certainly on a purely professional level the more one understands and knows about the history of science, the more cautious one becomes concerning the miraculous possibilities of medicine, and the humbler one becomes in relationship to the awesomeness and complexity of the species – homo sapiens. Anger at lack of knowledge or condemnation for ineffectual medicine plays no part here. Concerning our personal nature we could say that increased self-knowledge leading to true imagery of self is a humbling experience, because its aim is self-honesty. Knowledge of self consists in eliminating all necessary deceptions. Thus Neville (1978, p.53) concludes, 'self-knowledge in the pursuit of sagacity is not mere inquiry but the uncovering of deception. A sage is someone who at the very least knows the trickery of his heart'.

In the past nursing has undertaken to analyse its deceptions and values, (*see* Brykczynska, 1993), possibly entirely out of a desire to appear academically critical and questioning. This approach, which is quite appropriate for inanimate objects, such as art or research findings, or of thoughts such as ideologies or bodies of knowledge, is not appropriate, however, when practised in relation to innermost drives, ambitions and inclinations, i.e. personal values. To simply unmask 'the trickery of the heart' of nursing is possibly indicative of entirely missing the point. This is not to say that at the 'heart' of nursing one finds nothing but good and positive values – for it would be very strange if mortal women (and men) managed to arrange their affairs such that their 'minds move in charity, rest in providence, and turn upon the poles of truth', as Bacon (1972, p.4), would say. Rather, unmasking the trickery of the heart of the profession shows up how truly human and entirely vulnerable we are; how dependent on our historically fashioned and socio-culturally and physiologically determined nature our professional life really is.

Professional humility stems from understanding the true nature of our professional weaknesses, which in turn gives us the beginnings of an acquired wisdom.

If we ourselves also pursue a determined policy of self-knowledge in the aim of achieving a true picture of ourselves, we can also become wise; but we do not live in isolation, and images of ourself are painted by colours and strokes determined by time and place. Neville (1978) sees the need for the 'sages' to understand the world around them, for sages 'understand the combinations and ambiguities of these (emotions and events) in the lives of persons and in the affairs of peoples, and their understanding allows them so to follow the trail of what is important through the underbrush of triviality that they cleave to what is essential' (p. 54). The ultimate aim of the wise person is to know what it is essential to know, while everything else, all other knowledge, strictly speaking, is trivia. Wisdom depends on discernment of those facts that are essential and those that constitute fanciful digressions. Knowing when the fanciful digression is the heart of the matter constitutes the nature of true wisdom, a fact as much appropriate to the sagacious individual as to an entire professional body. It does not need much explanation that what constitutes 'knowledge' for one individual may seem trivia to another, and what is seen as essential for one discipline may be marginalized by another. These shifts in essential emphasis add to the colour and vibrancy of public life, and constitute the essence of creative strife.

In a particular profession, however, there would be an expectancy of some shared, common values concerning what would be considered essential knowledge; these would be collectively recognized and acknowledged by the professionals concerned (*see* Brykczynska, 1993). There would be a sense of collective professional discernment and wisdom based on shared knowledge.

According to Neville (1978), a sage is a person who understands people. This is a similar claim made on many nurses, for a sage 'grasps not only the nature and structure of affairs in the world, but also the way these affairs are felt in the subjectives lives of those who participate in them' (p.54). Understanding people is what many nurses consider as part of their professional *raison d'etre*; thus, psychiatric nurses would claim that it is essential knowledge for them, and health visitors may say that it is precisely understanding people that enables them to successfully influence the health patterns of their clients. Neville (1978) points out, however, that a sages' understanding of the world and people in it is fundamentally different to the understanding shared by the 'un'-wise. Most significantly, sages, whom he considers to be no 'fools', base their understanding of people more on processed, reflective, experiential exposure to incidents, rather than to an intuitive conditioning. Thus he points out, 'sages focus on the connections of life, on the meanings and consequences of things. Meanings and connections are no less matters of feeling than emotions. But they are learned from long experience, not from intuitive encounters. Sages must live through events in order to understand their texture' (p.54). This argument has been well addressed by those in nursing who wish that nurses would express more empathy in working with patients.

If a wise person understands people from a perspective of self-knowledge, where knowledge of one's true image induces a personal humility, this facilitates seeing the other in the same unfrivolous and unflattering light and thereby enables the making of true and correct connections between life events and the 'meaning of things'. One might well start to consider what does this understanding of the nature of wise people tell us about the nature of wise nurses? How would a wise nurse differ from a foolish nurse or even merely a knowledgeable nurse, or is there no perceptive difference between them? It is possible that, if no differences are perceived, a strictly pragmatic approach to the nature of wisdom in professional life might yield greater analytical returns. One detail that repeatedly crops up in the philosophical and psychological literature pertaining to wisdom that is not necessarily taken up by academics and other professionals, such as nurses, refers to the observation noted by Aristotle, two and half thousand years ago, that wisdom takes time to develop. Wise people must, as Neville points out, 'live through events in order to understand their textures', (p.54), and living through events takes time. Now obviously life can construe our fates in such a way that wisdom can be gained at an unsuspectingly early age, but this is usually at a very high emotional price. The processing and reflection on life's events have been artificially condensed. There has been no let-up in the 'amount' of life-events to be processed, only an increase of intensity of experiences over a shorter period of time. Just as one can savour and delight in a good cognac all evening, so one can drink it down in one gulp. The same brandy, and possibly the same or similar sensory reactions, but one approach to drinking gives time for reflection on the taste, while the other method of drinking gives one minimal time for reflection and therefore is harder to achieve. In practice one may see a young child gain much wisdom if it is exposed to many life-events requiring much reflection on its part, e.g. if the child had developed cancer. An adult normally would need to live a long life, especially if it were an uneventful life, to reach the same insights as a young child battling with childhood leukaemia for five or six years. We tend to think, on the whole, of the wise person as someone who has lived at least a bit longer than ourselves, for wisdom is seen as the fruit of a reflective and long life. To the extent that experienced nurses reflect on their professional life they too can be seen to be wise. Landmark works of Benner (1984), in North America, and the insights captured by Pam Smith (1992) in the United Kingdom, beautifully emphasize this point.

I would hazard to say that most professional nurses can think of at least one or two living examples of wise nursing colleagues, and it would be paradise on earth if one of those wise nurse-colleagues were also known to us personally in the capacity of a mentor and professional companion. The degree to which we have difficulties, however, in naming such an identifiable wise nurse, who should also be our mentor, indicates the degree to which professional inadequacy exists within our profession. Therefore, before we turn to point the finger of blame for our professional strife outside our profession, and start blaming others for its shortcomings and problems, let us first consider how to foster more wise nurses among our own ranks.

It was the wise, altruistic physician Albert Schweitzer who said that in order to ascribe to a notion of progress and civilization it was necessary to manifest hope and think optimistically, for 'we become workers for that universal, spiritual and material progress which we call civilization only in so far as we affirm that the world and life possess some sort of meaning, or which is the same thing, only in so far as we think optimistically' (Schweitzer, 1961 p.7). A discouraged, pessimistic profession, full of disheartened practitioners, can neither provide innovation in the art of nursing nor meaningfully contribute to an improvement in health-care 'civilization'.

Needless to say, it is not easy to be optimistic about oneself, one's future and one's profession, to care sufficiently to develop a virtue of wisdom. The question remains, however, how does one encourage the development of wisdom? Albert Schweitzer (1961) considers that an understanding of moral values contributes to an increased understanding of self and promotes a society conducive to re-socialization; thus 'it is only in his struggle to become ethical that man comes to possess real value as a personality' (p.6) – a statement reminiscent of Neville's analysis of the self-knowledge required of the wise person. For Schweitzer (1961), individual members of society need to become 'ethical' if a change is to be brought to society as a whole, because 'it is only under the influence of ethical convictions that the various relations of human society are formed in such a way that individuals and peoples can develop in an ideal manner' (p.6). It is the moral development of individual members of society that will help in turn to foster a societal climate conducive to moral growth and individualization of nurses. In summary, as we have already shown, the contemporary individual can become a wise person through the combined and overlapping aspects of personal development, as the habitual enactment of virtue suggested by Aristotle, or through the cultivation of intellectual abilities tempered with humour and gentleness, as demonstrated by female medieval scholastics, or through the appropriate understanding of an utilization of scientific knowledge, as proposed by philosophers of science, and lastly through an analysis and understanding of self that is based on constructive, hope-filled moral insights as illustrated by Neville (1978). For Schweitzer (1961) the most elemental factor in all of these approaches was the cultivation of an ethical foundation for our civilization (and society) because he felt that even if all the other elements of the equation were in place, without an ethical foundation, civilization itself would collapse and all our efforts with it. This observation is certainly worth reflecting upon, considering some of the technical and materialistic, especially scientific, progresses we are currently witnessing, but which seem devoid of wisdom, that is, a sense of the 'ethical', such as artificially maintaining pregnancies in post-menopausal women (Blain, 1993).

Yet we need not look towards other disciplines to consider whether lack of moral development is one of the causes of our professional distress where otherwise we should be looking at the golden era of nursing arts and sciences. How else can we explain the record number of complaints against nurses? Complaints range from accusations of physical and sexual abuse of patients, upon occasion even manslaughter, through to lack of cultivation of skills and abilities, e.g. by performing tasks for which one is not adequately prepared, or by inadequate communication with patients and their families resulting in hurt, misunderstanding and lack of consideration for the public common weal. This last is evidenced by such anti-social behaviour as persistent unexplained non-attendance at work, theft from the workplace or general under-performance at work as a result of working two jobs where one job is done at night. Such anti-social and potentially dangerous behaviour even in our present climate of job insecurity is extremely common and probably reflects a total sense of professional burn-out. To what extent the behaviour probably reflects existant ills and societal woes, more than contributory causes of health-care unrest, is not clear. The moral cycle whereby moral agents influence society, which in turn produces a particular type of morally creative health care system that can then foster or discourage an ethical approach appropriate for its nurses, becomes evident. The question to which we must therefore return is, how can we break the potential for negativity inherent in the present social system and start producing wise nurses who can be seen to care and seen to be the creatively active, knowledgeable, moral agents of society?

Nursing is a professionalised form of caring, it is the realization in practice of wisdom and compassion, where caring has as its prime focus the maintenance, restoration and intervention in matters of health (Brykczynska, 1992a, 1992b). Nurses approach the client or patient from a perspective of knowledgeable health-centred caring; knowledge about health-care matters influences the nature of caring and caring about health-care matters shapes the domain of nursing knowledge. There is then a symbiotic relationship between the acquired wisdom of the profession (its reflective knowledge base) and expressions of compassion, where compassion is the affective expression of nurses' caring concern for their patients' welfare. Thus, wisdom needs compassion to achieve its full expression, an expression witnessed every time a nurse sensitively and appropriately intervenes on the behalf of a patient or client. If nurses are to increase their reflective professional knowledge and thereby also self-knowledge in the pursuit of wisdom, they need also to look at the concept of professional compassion. By analysing the nature of nursing compassion they will also determine the nature of the relationship itself, between wisdom and compassion.

Primo Levi, the Italian writer who spent the latter part of the Second World War in a Nazi concentration camp, reflects in his autobiographical account of the experience upon the utter creative (yet totally compassionate) waste of energies expressed by the mothers of children in the transit camp (1969). He notes that mothers prepared food for the journey, washed the children and packed the luggage, and that at dawn of the day when they would be heading towards the 'East', the 'barbed wire was full of children's washing hung out in the wind to dry. Nor did they forget the diapers, the toys, the cushions and the hundred other small things which mothers remember and which children always need . . .' (p.7). A mother's compassion is undoubtedly partly intuitive, as no-one tells a mother to remember the nappies. For the nurse, before compassion can become totally internalized and intuitive, this ability to see the need for creative intervention in the welfare of a stranger must be nurtured and a deliberate program of socio-cultural–behavioural and moral development instituted. In professional language we would talk about a particular educational approach.

This educational approach is a conscious attempt by leaders of the profession and educationalists to transmit relevant knowledge and values to the aspiring nurse, so that she or he will be in a position to act compassionately, out of a 'taught' intuition. The profession tries to share some of its acquired wisdom.

Wisdom processes life events and renders them susceptible to the influence of compassion, which is maybe why wise mothers will continue to care for their children in the face of adversity; they will express intuitive compassion based on a natural home-spun wisdom. Levi (1969) observes that 'If you and your child were going to be killed tomorrow, would you not give him to eat today?' (p.7), an observation that would also come naturally to wise nurses working in palliative care, as they wash and set the hair of a woman whose living days are numbered. It is wisdom that discerns when and how to intervene, it is compassion that has the means to express that wisdom. Moreover, it is not just selected individuals who are capable of combining wisdom and compassion, to deliver perfect care. Care, the result of perfect interaction between wisdom and compassion, can be demonstrated by anybody, a salutary reminder to nurses that caring is not and can never be their sole prerogative. This does not mean however, that true nursing can occur without or in spite of, caring (*see* Brykczynska, 199a, 1992 b). Neither is nursing, of course, the sole prerogative of professionally qualified, registered individuals who are legally entitled to call themselves 'professional nurses'. The history of humanity is replete with examples of caring, professional non-nurses, who have superbly and compassionately nursed strangers. These people have always demonstrated in their caring behaviour a creative combination of wisdom and compassion.

Once in the concentration camp, Primo Levi contracts typhus and finds himself in the sanitation 'hospital' block. There, owing to the wisdom and compassion of a small group of dedicated individuals (none of whom were physicians or health-care workers), such creative caring of sick inmates took place, that whereas in the neighbouring 'hospital blocks' the sick inmates were dying daily and left to rot unburied for no-one had the energy (or goodwill) to intervene, in his block, only one inmate died of the eleven on the ward prior to liberation. This 'care' of sick inmates was conducted in the most adverse of circumstances imaginable, and without the benefit of 'professional knowledge'. Levi (1969), observing one of his friends nurse a sick inmate, comments that he 'lifted him from the gound with the tenderness of a mother, cleaned him as best as possible with straw taken from the mattress and lifted him into the remade bed in the only position in which the unfortunate fellow could lie' (p.137). If this description is not the picture of dedicating nursing I suggest we either look for a new definition of nursing or re-evaluate our present approach to patients. What makes this description of nursing so poignant is that there was no shade of 'professionalism' or self-interest, even of species-preservation. For even though some of the actions of the dedicated nucleus of self-styled 'nurses' were undertaken to help curb the spread of the disease, this was only a small part of the story. It would have been possible to curtail the spread of disease (as they obviously managed to do) without expressing 'tenderness' and pro-active concerns. That this caring came at a particularly high cost was not lost on the sick, bed-ridden onlookers who saw what it took in the form of energy and willpower to express such otherly love. Levi (1969) continues 'I judged his self-sacrifiice by the tiredness which I would have had to overcome in myself to do what he had done' (p.137). An eloquent definition of empathy and compassion.

Caring, the result of wisdom and compassion, does not come easily, but when it is present it not only creatively benefits the object of its attention, but also in a positive feedback mechanism spurs the carer on to continue caring and inspires hope in the cared for. Bruno Bettelheim (1991), the Jewish child-psychologist, who also survived the trauma of a concentration camp, notes that caring spurs on to more caring and in itself is energizing – 'This helping and being helped raised the spirits' (p.138). Like Primo Levi, he sees a connection between the courage it takes to do good even in a concentration camp, i.e. to demonstrate wisdom and compassion in the form of caring, and the unusually high cost it may involve. Thus, it was not a cheap glorification of self that changed a prisoner into a hero. Escapees from concentration camps were not automatic heroes, however 'daring and brilliant' their escape; for it meant death, torment, and increased distress to the remainder of the prisoners – that is, one person's freedom came at the cost of many more lives, from among those left behind. The price of freedom in this context was socially and more importantly, ethnically, unacceptable. Courage and heroism were seen only in those individuals who disinterestedly cared for others, at a personal cost. In fact, Bettelheim suggests they actually had to lose a sense of personal hope (that is, gain, even survival) to become 'liberated' enough to be able to truly care for the stranger, in what must be seen as one of the most inhospitable and non-caring environments ever constructed by man. Thus he comments, 'Once they abandoned hope for their personal existence, it became easier for them to act heroically, and help others' (p.138). Compassion demonstrated by these men and women came at an extraordinarily high price, which is why we look at them as heroes or as role models, if somewhat reluctantly. As Bettelheim (1991), concludes, 'Heroism can be the highest assertion of individuality . . . only those who suffered for their efforts to protect other prisoners were accepted as heroes' (p.139).

At this stage, the nurse may well ask, what must she do to promote wisdom and compassion, in order to be able to care disinterestedly? Must she equate her place of work with the horrors of a concentration camp, and heroically ignoring her own survival instincts, throw herself into the promotion of care of patients, at a personal risk of burn-out and utter frustration? Such a scenario would be both absurd and highly dangerous. Absurd, because it ignores the reality of wisdom – which if nothing else, is the very opposite of foolhardy impetuous stances, and dangerous because it taunts the system into accepting a reality that is incompatible with nature. Nurses are not asked to nurse in 'un-nurseable' environments, but they are asked to humanize the inhumane environment and make it receptive to their 'caring mode of being' (Roach, 1984). This undoubtedly takes a certain amount of wisdom and compassion; as Bettelheim (1991) noted in regards to the nature of caring, 'the success or failure of any mass society will depend on whether or not a man reshapes his personality so he can modify the society into one that is truly human; in our case, into one where we are not coerced by technology, but bend it to our human needs . . .' (p.268). Nurses must be in control of their environments if they wish to deliver a humanizing care in spite of technology and societal conditions. Their care must bend the environment to the needs of patients.

It is interesting, therefore, to note, that just as for philosophers, theologians and writers, so for Bettelheim, the 'wise' psychologist, changes in society start from endeavours to re-shape the personality of the moral agent. Rather than trying to re-shape society, or influence central funding of the National Health System, or change the pattern of working practices within the health-care field, philosophers, writers, wise psychologists and 'enlightened' counsellors all appear to be advising a turn towards the cultivation of personal wisdom. They are saying that by a concerted effort at self-knowledge, a pursuit of virtue, a concern for the other and love of scholarship, the ensuing wisdom that will be cultivated will increase the natural concommitant compassion and put into its rightful perspective that which troubles and surrounds us. With the acquisition of wisdom, life's problems will reflect a new set of priorities. Wisdom will then be able to determine how concern for the other, through compassion, needs to be manifested.

Perhaps the most insightful question that needs to be finally addressed, but that cannot ever be fully answered on behalf of another, is to what extent nurses really want to be 'wise'. In an age of quick solutions, easy answers, fast remedies, and market economies, everything speaks against the acquisition of wisdom, and with it, of a wise compassion. All the sages and wise counsellors down the ages have emphasized the benefits that come to the individual and thereby to society by cultivating wisdom, but they also have emphasized the time involved, the personal cost in energy and total engrossment and the potential price to pay for some, in a predominantly still pre-sagacious society, that may well feel threatened by the Wise and Compassionate. One cannot legislate that all qualified nurses be wise, for that is beyond the powers of legislative bodies, but, as the nursing authorities have attempted to do, they can urge and provide directives as to how they would like to see nurses behave and act. The recommendation for the modern nurse is to be a 'reflective practitioner', one who reflects on a wholesome practice. This reflection on practice is nothing else but an analysis borne in wisdom on the demonstration of compassion.

It was Aristotle, the archetypical sage, who in his book on Metaphysics commented that, 'as owls' eyes are at noonday, so is our mental vision blind to what in its own nature is the most evident of all' (Aristotle, 1952 p.35). Most evident of all, to those in nursing, is that reflective caring is based on wisdom and compassion. The symbiosis of wisdom and compassion is as strong as nuclear particles in an atom. Like the constituents of an atom, to cleave the two apart spells disaster and distorts the original nature of things. Just as an unwise nurse will exhaust herself with misdirected compassion, it will not, therefore, be compassion that guides her work but pity, so a wise but uncompassionate nurse will be a contradiction in terms.

The ideal reflective practitioner, as promoted by Shön (1983) and others, is the wise and compassionate nurse, one who is the embodiment of disinterested professional caring.

REFERENCES

Aristotle *Metaphysics* (1952). University of Michigan Press, Ann Arbor.
Aristotle *Nichomachean Ethics* (1962). Bobbs Merrill, Indianapolis.
Bacon, F. (1973) *Essays*. Dent, London.
Benner, P. (1984) *From Novice to Expert*. Addison–Wesley, Menlo Park.
Bettelheim, B. (1991) *The Informed Heart*. Penguin, Harmondsworth.
Blain, S. (1993) Ova the Hill? *Nursing Standard*, 8(11), 46.
Brykczynska, G. (1992a) Caring: a dying art? In *Nursing Care: The Challenge to Change*. Jolley, M. and Brykczynska, G. (Eds), pp.1-45. Edward Arnold, London
Brykczynska, G. (1992b) Caring: some philosophical and spiritual reflections. In *Nursing Care: The Challenge to Change*. Jolley, M. and Brykczynska, G. (Eds), pp.225–61. Edward Arnold, London.

Brykczynska, G. (1993) Values in nursing: nightmares and nonsense. In *Nursing: Its Hidden Agendas*. Jolley, M. and Brykczynska, G. (Eds). Edward Arnold, London.

Bullock, A. and Stallybrass, O. (Eds) (1977) *The Fontana Dictionary of Modern Thought*. Fontana, London.

Evasdaughter, E. N. (1989) Julian of Norwich. In Waithe, M. E. (Ed). *A History of Women Philosophers*, Volume 2, pp.191-222. Klumer Academic Publishers, Dordrecht.

Foucault, M. (1972) *The Archaeology of Knowledge*. Tavistock, London.

Jolley, M. (1989) The professionalisation of nursing: the uncertain path. In Jolley, M. and Allan, P. (Eds). *Current Issues in Nursing*, pp.1–22. Chapman and Hall, London.

Kuhn, T. (1962) *The Structure of Scientific Revolutions*. University of Chicago Press, Cambridge.

Levi, P. (1969) *If This is a Man*. New English Library, London.

Lloyd, E. A. (1968) *Aristotle: The Growth and Structure of his Thought*. Cambridge University Press, Cambridge.

Murdoch, I. (1962) *Metaphysics as a Guide to Morals*. Chatto and Windus, London.

Neville, R. (1978) *Soldier, Sage, Saint*. Fordham University Press, New York.

Plato (1974) *The Republic*. Penguin, Harmondsworth.

Polanyi, M. (1962) *Personal Knowledge: Towards a Post Critical Philosophy*. Routledge and Kegan Paul, London.

Polanyi, M. and Prosch, H. (1975) *Meaning*. University of Chicago Press, Chicago.

Popper, K. (1972) *Objective Knowledge*. Oxford University Press, Oxford.

Roach, S. (1984) *Caring: The Human Mode of Being: Implications for Nursing Perspectives in Caring, Monograph 1*. Faculty of Nursing, University of Toronto, Toronto.

Russell, B. (1967) *The Problems of Philosophy*. Oxford University Press, Oxford.

Schilpp, P. A. (Ed) (1974) The Philosophy of Karl Popper. *The Library of Living Philosophers*, Vol XIV Book 1/ Book 2. The Open Court Publishing Co, La Salle, Illinois.

Schon, D. A. (1983) *The Reflective Practitioner: How Professionals Think in Action*. Basic Books, New York City.

Schweitzer, A. (1961) *The Decay and the Restoration of Civilization*. Unwin, London.

Shorter Oxford English Dictionary (1973) Third Edition. Clarendon Press, Oxford.

Smith, P. (1992) *The Emotional Labour of Nursing*. Macmillan, Basingstoke.

Upjohn, S. (1992) *All Shall Be Well*. Darton, Longman and Todd, London.

Waithe, M. E. (Editor) (1989) *A History of Women Philosophers, Volume 2: 500–1600 AD*. Klumer Academic, Dordrecht.

Zedler, B. H. (1989) Marie le Jars de Gournay. In Waithe, M E (Ed) *A History of Women Philosophers*, Volume 2, pp.285–307. Klumer Academic Publishers, Dordrecht.

2.

NEW WINE IN OLD BOTTLES?

INTRODUCTION ('THE WINE CELLAR')

The past two decades have witnessed a continuing movement towards reform in both pre- and post-registration nursing education. Change is now almost a constant companion for us all. This chapter will explore the nature and impact of those reforms on both pre- and post-registration education. The use of vinous metaphors will be used sparingly throughout the text in an attempt to enhance the chapter's 'flavour'. First, the problems associated with apprenticeship models of pre-registration nursing education in relation to dominant curriculum ideologies will be highlighted. This will be followed by an account of the setting up of Project 2000 pre-registration programmes (the nouveau Beaujolais metaphor) and the progress of some of the demonstration schemes with reference to available research.

Following the exploration of pre-registration education, attention will be directed towards reforms in post-registration education, focussing on CATS (Credit Accumulation and Transfer Schemes) and the modularization of courses (the mixed case metaphor).

Finally, the evolving role of teachers of nurses, health visitors and midwives in the context of the current educational reforms will be addressed (the Dom Perignon metaphor).

A critical perspective will be adopted throughout the chapter, concluding with an overall assessment of the 'vintage' of the reforms.

THE PAST ('OLD BOTTLES')

Scrimshaw (1983) describes four different curriculum ideologies, i.e. classical/liberal humanism, instrumentalism, progressivism and reconstructionism. The nature and relative merits of each of these ideologies will now be examined alongside their related four ordering principles of curriculum construction, i.e. maps of key subjects, schedules of essential skills, portfolios of meaningful student experiences, and agendae of important cultural issues. This will provide a brief socio-historical context to events leading up to the current educational reforms.

Curricula based on classical/liberal humanism are essentially knowledge-centred courses, i.e. courses based on maps of key subjects (Beattie, 1987). This can be regarded as one of the oldest approaches to curriculum planning and reflected most of the early approaches to nurse training, with curricula containing 'bins' of anatomy and physiology, pathology and microbiology, medical and surgical nursing and other topics. To be fair, many of the topics could be described as 'appellation contrôllée' subjects, but many were not very palatable 'bin ends' – for example, the workings of sewage farms!

An instrumental curriculum can be described as competency-centred. This can also be described as a means-to-an-end model of curriculum, with the objectives or learning outcomes the means to reach the ends (aims) of the course. Beattie (1987) describes this ordering principle as a schedule of basic skills, but the writer prefers the term'essential' rather than basic, since the latter tends to connote simple, whereas essential connotes fundamental. The General Nursing Council for England and Wales (GNC) and the Joint Board of Clinical Nursing Studies (JBCNS) both advocated the use of behavioural objectives in pre- and post-registration courses respectively for much of the 1960s.

However, humanistic psychology began to exert a strong influence on the delivery of nursing care and nursing education during the 1970s. Consequently, nurse teachers developed their courses on progressivist (i.e. more student-centred) ideologies of education. A good example of this was the revised 1982 syllabus for the initial first level preparation of mental health nurses and its implementation based on students' agendae and experiential learning. This approach clearly reflected Beattie's concept of the curriculum as a portfolio of meaningful experiences.

Whichever the dominant curriculum ideology, James and Jones (1992) explain how throughout history it has been necessary to change and develop the education of nurses, midwives and health visitors in order to meet the health care needs of society. This can be described as a predominantly reconstructionist approach to curriculum development and innovation, i.e. an approach that centres on the needs of society and in this example the consumers of health care (all of us at various times in our life). The relative merits of each curriculum-ordering principle and ideology can be summarized as follows:

1. Curriculum as a map of key subjects – (ordering principle)
    Ideology: liberal humanism
Positive aspects
• students need to be acquainted with a rapidly growing body of knowledge
• integration can be achieved by using interdisciplinary themes, e.g. the lifespan
• it is helpful to curriculum planners to refer to comprehensive subject maps
Negative aspects
• obsolete subject maps
• little integration of subject matter
• collection code curriculum (described later in the chaper)

2. Curriculum as a schedule of essential skills – (ordering principle)
    Ideology: instrumentalism
Positive aspects
• enables explicit communication between students, teachers and outside bodies
• explicit terms of reference for assessment provided
• specification of essential skills is important where areas of practical skill are
    deemed essential

• provides students with guides for self-directed learning

Negative aspects
• may be inflexible
• may be counter-intuitive
• may trivialize educational process
• students and teachers accountable to a utilitarian/instrumental mode of
    management/supervision

3. Curriculum as a portfolio of meaningful experiences – (ordering principle)
    Ideology: progressivism

Positive aspects
• locus of control with students
• humanistic ethos
• basis for action research
• critical incidents can provide the basis for experiential learning
• students have ownership of curriculum
• compatible with the tenets of adult education

Negative aspects
• unpredictable
• teachers may feel unprepared
• possible logistical problems
• 'patchy' coverage of key subjects

4. Curriculum as an agenda of important cultural issues – (ordering principle)
    Ideology: reconstructionism

Positive aspects
• topical issues addressed
• up-to-date currciulum
• wider socio-political context of health care provision addressed

Negative aspects
• issues may dominate the curriculum at the expense of other important curricular
    areas

(adapted from Beattie, 1987).

Many of the older traditional nurse curricula were founded on liberal humanism
and instrumentalism based on an apprenticeship model of training.

The problems of this model have been well documented (Judge, 1985) and a
detailed account will not be repeated here. However, it is worth being reminded
of some of the key problems associated with traditional nurse training
programmes:

• procedural and task-orientation rather than person-orientation
• the education needs of the students were often sacrified for the exigencies of
    the service

- unnecessary repetition of clinical experiences in order to fulfil workforce
    planning needs
- inadequate supervision of nurse learners in placement areas exacerbated by
    those students being counted as part of the workforce
- decline in popularity of careers in nursing in the face of other more attractive
    options (exacerbated by the anticipated decline in the number of school-
    leavers)

Prior to implementation of Project 2000 it should be stressed that many colleges of nursing had developed excellent pre-registration courses based on more progressive ideologies with a focus on health rather than disease. The availability of masters degrees in education and the increasing emphasis on curriculum studies in nurse teacher preparation courses have had a significant impact on the quality of submission documents. Many nurse teachers have moved away from single-minded curriculum approaches and have become much more creative in the development of both pre- and post-registration courses. This observation is founded on the writer being involved in numerous validation events for the English National Board, the Council for National Academic Awards (CNAA) and the University of Manchester. However, having gone through all that developmental work, colleges were now faced with having to devise Diploma level courses, with very tight deadlines for the submission of the documentation for validation purposes.

PROJECT 2000 ('A NEW VINTAGE')

In the summer of 1984 the United Kingdom Central Council (UKCC) established Project 2000, its aim being to 'determine the education and training required for the professional practice of nursing, midwifery and health visiting in relation to the projected health care needs in the 1990s and beyond and to make recommendations'.

In 1988 the Chairperson of the UKCC, Audrey Emerton, expressed the aims of the Project 2000 strategy. Its aims were to:

- provide the levels and types of nursing necessary for the future and which
            Government plans and health authorities' strategies demand
- reflect the principal aspirations of the professions to provide better care
- prove to be more cost effective in the medium term
- maintain the pre-eminent position of British nursing in the world
- address issues of finance and manpower realistically
(James and Jones, 1992).

The education and training reforms focused on the creation of a single level of practitioner. This 'vintage practitioner' was given the name of 'knowledgeable doer' and in the writer's view should at least have the following characteristics:

- be educated to diploma or degree level
- be able to transfer knowledge and skills to a range of health-care situations
- be able to assess client need and deliver individualized health care based on
     appropriate research if available
- manage change effectively through innovation and/or adaptation
- be a reflective practitioner
- be committed to their own continuing education and professional
     development

Evaluation of Project 2000 ('the wine tasters')

In April 1989 the Department of Health (DoH) commissioned the National Foundation for Education Research (NFER) to carry out an independent evaluation of the initial implementation phase of Project 2000. This evaluation consisted of six in-depth case studies from the thirteen demonstration districts for the project. Initially the research project was financed to run from February 1989 to September 1992, the latter date being when the first Project 2000 cohorts were set to complete their courses. The Research Advisory Group urged the DoH to extend the project until March 1993. It was considered essential that the evaluation should continue and include data on the effect the diplomates had on practice. The writer suggests that caution should be exercised in making judgements on the effectiveness of these practitioners too prematurely. Experienced wine tasters will explain that many good wines are reticent with their flavours and either need longer in the bottle or a little contact with oxygen to 'bring them out' (an interesting metaphor in the context of Project 2000 diplomates perhaps?).

The evaluation was carried out by two full-time researchers based at the NFER in Slough and two researchers with a part-time commitment to the project based in the NFER's northern office at the University of York.

Purpose of NFER Study
The purpose of the NFER study was to evaluate the intentions, processes, and outcomes of the six Project 2000 pilot schemes (Leonard & Jowett, 1990). It was intended that the evaluation would illuminate many of the issues raised by the educational reforms. The outcomes of the pilot schemes were considered to be especially important. Would these knowledgeable doers epitomize the well-informed and competent 'guardians' of the future of the nursing profession that were envisaged or would the metaphor of 'old wine in new bottles' prove true?

A longitudinal approach was adopted to enable the researchers to monitor the changing perceptions of key participants, e.g. the students, their teachers and colleagues from practice settings. The research design was very much of the naturalistic paradigm, which seeks to discover, describe, decode, translate and get to grips with the meaning of the social world (Jowett, 1992). A positivist approach was rejected as being inappropriate for this research since it aimed to deal with the complexities of different individuals interacting with one another in educational settings. Essentially the researchers were attempting to 'tease out' the embeddedness of social truths, a key tenet of naturalistic research. The researchers used a wide range of data collection methods, which included:

• questionnaires to the students
• interviews with the students
• interviews with course teachers and practice-based staff
• scrutiny of course documentation and other relevant written information
• assembly of comparative data
• interviews with other relevant professionals
• follow-up interviews

The Research Advisory Group felt that the profession could benefit from the preliminary findings of the research and recommended that a number of working papers should be disseminated. Valuable lessons from the research could be learned by those colleges in the throes of or on the threshold of their own Project 2000 implementation. A number of studies were undertaken concurrently with the NFER study, and many have followed since, and some with contentious findings. However, the findings of the NFER study, which were in the main quite positive, can be summarized as follows:

1. Planning issues
The quote which for the writer best sums up this aspect is from one of the respondents, who said: 'planning for the new course was like laying the lines while the train is coming' (Payne *et al*, 1991).

This epitomizes the tension that often occurs between curriculum maintenance and curriculum development. The former is concerned with managing a college's existing courses, e.g. non-Project-2000 pre-registration programmes and other post-registration courses. The latter is concerned with new initiatives which are often of a pressing nature.

Nurse teachers across all the districts commented on the pressure exerted by the rushed planning and implementation of the new programme. In such situations, as the writer has found, one is faced with sacrificing some of the normally sound principles of curriculum planning on the 'altar of expediency'. An example of this would be not involving all the key participants in the development of the course philosophy, which can lead to a lack of ownership.

In summary of this aspect, there was generally a lack of information dissemination about the new courses.

2. Curriculum planning
As previously mentioned, many colleagues had already developed their curricula on a health rather than disease-oriented model with shifts from medical to nursing models. The writer feels that at this point it is worth mentioning the much-maligned medical model. Continually lambasting the medical model is not helpful and is not in the spirit of interprofessional collegiality. Both the medical and nursing professions can learn much from each other and work in harmony for the

welfare of clients. Another problem was that many teachers were concerned about insufficient consultation between their colleagues resulting in some disjointedness and duplication of effort (Payne *et al*, 1991).

3. Teaching

The very large numbers associated with Project 2000 intakes compared to the 'traditional' courses have had quite an impact on teaching methods. Over the past decade, courses that prepare nurse teachers have concentrated very much on the development of a broad range of experiential methods. Many teaching staff were concerned that the skills they had learned on their teacher preparation courses would not now be fully exploited (Payne *et al*, 1991). In the writer's experience of visiting several colleges of nursing, although much had been invested in improving the facilities in lecture theatres, nevertheless 'performing' in front of large groups was said to be a daunting prospect by many nurse teachers.

The NFER researchers found another major concern among nurse teachers regarding the lack of time they had available for students. This the writer feels is becoming of increasing concern to nearly all teachers trying to cope with the large increase in student numbers across the education sector and the changing nature of assignment work, e.g. many more students are now undertaking research dissertations requiring supervision and co-supervision. The latter group come from students undertaking honours degree programmes following first level registration where research projects are a key aspect of level three academic work.

4. Management of change

This aspect of the research will be discussed with reference to the writer's adapted model of Bolam (1975) (cited English National Board for Nursing, Midwifery and Health Visiting, 1987). This model describes five interrelated factors to be considered when managing change, i.e. the innovation, the users, the locus of change, the change agent(s) and the change strategies and is depicted in the context of Project 2000 and the vinous metaphor in *Figure 1*.

Figure 1 The five interrelated factors involved when managing change

The innovation
(the wine)
Project 2000
demonstration schemes

The users
(the wine drinkers)
students
practice-based staff
managers
teachers

Loci of change
(the vineyards)
6 demonstration sites
including colleges of nursing,
higher education centres and
practice settings

Change agents
(the vintners)

Change strategies
(production and bottling)
(marketing and sales)

Curriculum developers ———————————— Combined strategy

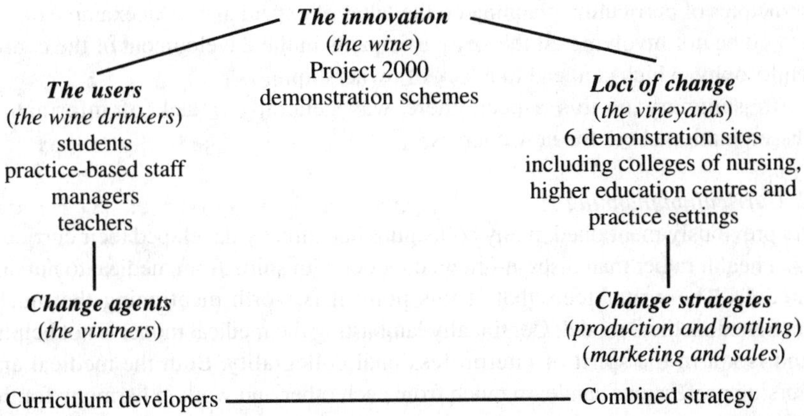

The innovation

A survey of the literature (particularly Rogers and Shoemaker, 1971 and English National Board for Nursing, Midwifery and Health Visiting, 1987) identified seven attributes that are correlated with the successful implementation of change. They will be used as a framework to discuss the innovation.

a) Relative advantage

This attribute is all about the relative merits of the proposed change over the status quo. The shortcomings of 'traditional' pre-registration nursing education schemes have been referred to earlier in the chapter. Project 2000 schemes have several advantages over their predecessors, e.g: full student rather than employee status, educationally led programmes, and enhancement of academic credibility with good advanced standing for entry into degree courses.

One relative disadvantage found so far is that some students have not felt very competent to give 'hands-on' care because of the way that their learning experiences had been organised and the different role sets of Project 2000 students. This has been a major concern for the students, their teachers and the staff in practice settings. However, this appears to have been less of a problem for students once they had entered their respective branch programmes. This is no doubt due to the students having 'found their feet' after ending 18 months in the common foundation programmes and having subsequently entered their chosen specialist areas.

b) Compatibility

This refers to the extent to which this major innovation is accepted by and is compatible with the personnel affected. There is no doubt that the principles that underpin the Project 2000 programmes have been widely accepted as highly desirable. However, some students on non-Project 2000 schemes have been concerned that their own preparation is considered as having less value, with many feeling that their own educational needs have been subordinated to those of their Project 2000 colleagues. Many nurse teachers have also felt that maintaining the motivation of the students on non-project 2000 schemes has proved to be a challenge.

Some of the clinically-based staff have been unsure of the role of the 'new' students asking questions such as: 'What is it that you can actually do while you are here, e.g. can you take a blood pressure?'

Even though a number of strategies were adopted to prepare the practice-based staff for the arrival of the new students, for example study days on a range of topics such as supervision and assessment, it was inevitable that there would be problems associated with role-expectations in view of the short time scales for implementation of the schemes.

This problem should be ameliorated as role expectations become clearer and practice-based staff develop more confidence through increased knowledge and understanding of what the diploma schemes are all about. The proliferation of effective mentorship and clinical preceptorship schemes should also make a major contribution in this respect. Sessions on mentorship and clinical supervision are now regarded as an essential aspect of continuing professional education.

c) *Communicability*

This attribute is all about the relative ease of communicating about the means of the change. The concept of Project 2000 is in fact quite complex to communicate. It has several defining attributes eg diploma level course, supernumerary status, knowledgeable doer.

The concept of academic level in particular is in the writer's view not well-understood. This is partially due to a dearth of research in the area of academic levels and the variety of different interpretations of levels 1, 2, 3 and M. The writer proposes the following short descriptions of academic levels 1, 2, 3 and M, followed by a description of associated assessment criteria, identified in table one. This will then be followed by an example of how those criteria could be reflected in an academic essay on the management of pain:

Level 1

This level encompasses the fundamental knowledge and skills appropriate for professional practice. This involves analysis, problem-solving, decision-making and the application of theory to practice. Academic work at this level should fulfil at least the first six of the ten assessment criteria in table 1 to a satisfactory standard.

Level 2

This level involves the study of theory and practice at greater depth and breadth. This is achieved by an extension of knowledge and skills through the use of appropriate conceptual frameworks and research findings. This level is epitomised by synthesis and holistic understanding in addition to the features required at level 1. Academic work at this level should fulfil at least the first eight of the ten assessment criteria in table 1 to a satisfactory standard.

Level 3

This level encompasses all the level 1 and 2 attributes but is further characterised by critical evaluation and innovative thinking in an area of professional practice. Academic work at this level should fulfil all ten of the assessment criteria listed to a satisfactory standard.

Level M

This level is characterised by an autonomous and creative approach to professional practice. At this postgraduate level, students should attempt to extend the boundaries of knowledge and practice, by developing new theory to guide practice or new theory from innovative practice.

This level is also characterised by extended knowledge and skills in consultancy, education and research. Academic work at this level should fulfil all ten of the assessment criteria (shown in *Table 1*, overleaf) at a deeper level than the level 3 requirement.

Table 1 Assessment criteria for written academic work

1. There should be clear focus on the topic of the assignment, beginning with an outline of the approach taken and an indication of the context.
2. Relevant theory and related knowledge should be included.
3. Information should be supported from published sources and referenced correctly.
4. Knowledge should be applied appropriately with an indication of the relevance to practice.
5. The line of argument/discussion should be coherent and the assignment concluded appropriately.
6. There should be evidence of appropriate and up-to-date reading to support the arguments/discussion in breadth and depth.
7. There should be an awareness of the wider issues/implications of the assignment reflected in the assignment.
8. There should be evidence of an analytical/problem-solving approach to the assignment.
9. There should be critical evaluation of the ideas and material which includes independent comment.
10. Synthesis/innovative thinking should be a feature of the assignment.

(adapted from criteria used by the Institute of Advanced Nursing Education, 1992).

The writer suggests that the criteria provide students and assessors with guidelines for action, but as unqualified statements, may not be particularly helpful. For example, if a student is advised that his/her work does not reflect sufficient analysis and synthesis, what does this actually mean?

The following illustrations are intended to 'flesh out' the criteria and give some idea of what they mean in practice using an assignment title such as:

'Critically discuss the role of the nurse in the management of pain.'

1. Focus on topic, outlining approach and context
This sample introduction covers both elements of the above criterion, e.g: I will start by comparing and contrasting some different definitions of pain, followed by an outline of pain theories. The main emphasis will be on the nurse's role in the management of pain with reference to both pharmacological and non-pharmacological interventions. A review of different pain assessment tools will be included in this context. I will conclude by proposing the principles which should be included in a protocol for the management of pain.

2. Relevant theory/related knowledge
A matrix can help students to consider appropriate theory and related knowledge, to prioritize information, and to act as an aide-memoire for a summary. It can be extended/reduced as required provided that the inclusion of the content is relevant and appropriate. A word of caution is necessary here. Enthusiasm may lead to the

inclusion of too much content, thus sacrificing depth for quantity. The selection of content needs to be considered in the context of the assignment title and the word allowance. An example of a matrix might be:

Theory	Acute/chronic pain
nursing	model for care e.g. Orem
physiology	pain theories
psychology	perception of pain
sociology	cultural differences
pharmacology	analgesia
ethics	withholding analgesics

3. References

A modified Harvard system is the one most commonly used referencing system in British and American literature. Care must be taken to ensure that points/arguments are acknowledged/supported appropriately. If a system other than a modified Harvard is adopted, it should be used consistently.

4. Application and relevance

This is one of the most, if not the most important criterion. The matrix can be used here to good effect. Theory informs practice and practice can inform theory as follows:

theory

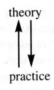

practice

Two of the writer's favourite questions are 'So what?' and 'What can I do on Monday?' The point I am trying to make here is instrumentalist in nature, e.g. what are the implications of cultural differences in the perception of pain for practice in different health-care settings?

5. Coherence and conclusion

A logical ordering of material is required here with reference to the planning matrix. The use of linking sentences can enhance the flow, such as 'having discussed x, attention will be focussed on y', e.g. having compared and contrasted different pain theories, attention will now be focused on some of the main psychological perspectives with reference to nursing research in this area.

In the conclusion, readers should be reminded of the main points (the matrix can help again here).

6. Breadth and depth of up-to-date and appropriate reading

It is important that there has been a comprehensive literature review, citing from primary sources whenever possible. Up-to-date source material should be included. An alphabetically indexed filing system is invaluable in this respect. The time it takes to write up the references and bibliography, often left to the last minute, should not be underestimated.

7. Wider issues/implications
This criterion invites students to include issues from the wider cultural agenda relevant to the main theme(s) of the assignment such as political and ethical issues, e.g. nurse prescribing and the use of complementary therapies.

8. Analysis/problem-solving
This is characterized by the ability to break down conceptual material into its component parts, and the separation of the the important aspects of information from the less important, e.g. discriminating between doctors' and nurses' roles in the management of pain.

9. Critical evaluation/independent comment
Independent comment can be differentiated from a purely anecdotal approach, e.g. Smith (1985) argued that 'x' was the most appropriate approach in the management of post-operative pain, but Jones (1987) refuted Smith's claims following her research into the area. However, I suggest that an adaptation of both strategies offers more scope because etc.

10. Synthesis/innovative thinking
Whereas analysis involves breaking down conceptual material into its component parts, synthesis requires that the various components are combined into a new whole. Creativity is present because something novel is produced, e.g. a discussion of the principles that could underpin a protocol for the management of pain.

It is essential that further research is carried out in the area of academic levels and associated criteria so that equity, fairness and commensuarability of decision-making with regard to assessment, credit recognition and accreditation can be effected. The change attribute of potential complexity will now be considered.

d) Complexity
This attribute is concerned with the relative ease of difficulty in the use of an innovation. Several logistical difficulties have arisen in the delivery of Project 2000 schemes, notably the 'bottlenecks' in some practical placements, particularly in the community. Other logistical difficulties have arisen in the case of multi-site colleges with students needing transportation to different sessions. Complexity also relates to levels of understanding of the nature of the change and its implementation and clearly that has been problematic as was mentioned under compatibility, i.e. confusion over exactly what roles Project 2000 students could fulfil during their practical placements. In terms of the complexity of Project 2000, the writer is reminded here of the distinction Docking (1987) makes between curriculum renewal and curriculum innovation. The former is concerned with changes to a system without a fundamental change in attitudes, whereas the latter is much more profound.

e) Trialability

This attribute is concerned with the possibility of piloting a change on either a small or large scale. Successful pilots can lead to a 'ripple' effect where a successful change in one group can lead to its implementation with another group. The early demonstration schemes can be seen as large pilot schemes and much has been learned to help others with their curriculum development and implementation.

f) Observability

This attribute is concerned with the actual visibility of an innovation. In the context of Project 2000, the increased size of the curriculum submission documents is notable.

g) Relevance

This attribute is concerned with the relevance of an innovation in a given situation and merits no further comment as this has been well covered earlier in the chapter.

The users

The users of Project 2000 include a wide range of personnel, in fact all those associated with non-diploma courses and many more besides, e.g. personnel in community settings not formerly involved. Reference has already been made to the effect this major innovation has had on nurse teachers and other education personnel. The pressure has been enormous in preparing substantive curriculum documents, negotiating placements and preparing for conjoint validation while at the same time managing their ongoing work.

Research into the students' feelings has revealed interesting data. Robinson (1992) found that the first group of students in her college had great difficulty in understanding the purpose of some of the early non-nursing placements. This problem was ameliorated by shortening those placements and making them more focused on specific content-related tasks. Many students were concerned about the lack of practical experience and their lack of proficiency in this respect, a concern shared by the qualified staff in those practice settings.

Much of the disenchantment and concern felt during the common foundation programmes eased on entry to the branches, which was both welcome and a relief for all concerned.

One of the main points of controversy of Project 2000 is the false perception amongst some critics that diploma courses will render the non-diploma courses almost worthless. However, the writer dismisses this assertion, feeling that there is room for every type of qualified nurse.

The loci of change

The loci of change are diverse in nature and spread nationally. Many organizational barriers had to be addressed. It is asserted that the main ones were:

• lack of understanding of how the relationship with institutions of higher
     education would affect nurse teachers' roles
• inadequate human and material resources

• too many other competing innovations being introduced at the same time, e.g.
   changes in the nature and delivery of post-registration education (discussed
   later in this chapter).

For a vineyard to produce a good vintage, a number of environmental
conditions need to co-exist, e.g. good soil, a disease-free vine, appropriate
fertilization and the right mixture of sun and rain. The same is true of a locus of
change for that change to flourish, and in this context an open environment with
good leadership, a conceptually sound curriculum, and quality staff to implement
the changes are pre- and co-requisites.

The change agents

The term change agent has four fundamental functions according to Jones (1969).
They are outlined from the perspectives of the college principal and designated
project leader in the context of Project 2000 as follows:

i)   To diagnose the problem, i.e. how to meet the curricular deadlines imposed
ii) To identify and clarify the goals of change, e.g. how to prepare a quality
         programme that is capable of efective translation into practice at the
         same time as meeting the requirements of validating bodies
iii) To develop strategies and tactics to introduce change, e.g. appointing/
         redeploying teaching staff to prepare the documentation and other
         personnel, such as the preparation of mentors and supervisors
iv) To establish and maintain a working relationship with change users

The responsibility that falls on principals and their project leaders cannot be
underemphasized. It is gratifying to know that they all felt the effort was worth it
(Jowett *et al*, 1991).

The change strategies

The writer suggests that three elements of the combined strategy described by
Sieber (1971) (cited Ketefian, 1978) appear to have been those most utilised by
change agents in the context of Project 2000, in that:

a) change agents, e.g. college principals, invested authority in their project
         leaders to see the curriculum innovations through to validation and
         beyond
b) curriculum development was based on a rational/problem-solving model
c) change agents endeavoured to seek consensus on new norms, e.g. in schemes
         of study, schemes of assessment, teaching/learning methodologies and
         practical placements

The fourth element of Sieber's combined strategy is concerned with two-way
communication and expertise in group processes. It is in this aspect, perhaps not
surprisingly, that there have been diverse experiences, many positive and many
quite negative. Buckenham (1992) reports how, in his college, staff felt alienated
and confused by the innovation. Communication problems have also been found

in many other sites (Jowett *et al*, 1991; Robinson, 1992). James and Jones (1992) allude to the compromises that have had to be made between political expediency and some aspects of professionalism. However, many examples of effective change strategies can be applauded, found both in the literature on Project 2000 and experienced by the writer on validation events.

To conclude this part of the chapter, the writer asks the question are Project 2000 students going to be distinctively 'better' nurses? It is a value-laden rhetorical question, I know. The writer is optimistic but suggests that the quality of the 'vintage' needs to be researched, which should prove to be most illuminating. As the writer suggested earlier, perhaps the 'wine' needs 'laying down' for a while before making too premature a judgement.

The 'nouveau beaujolais' will be left on the 'wine rack' for the time being. Attention will now be focused on some of the contents of a 'mixed case', starting with an overview of credit accumulation and transfer.

CREDIT ACCUMULATION AND TRANSFER

The emergence and proliferation of credit accumulation and transfer schemes (CATS) has had a major impact on the structure and provision of post-registration education for health care professionals. This is reflected in a number of ways, e.g:

• institutions developing frameworks for academic progression
• pathway development within frameworks
• tariffs for academic/professional qualifications with credit ratings
• accreditation processes and procedures
• intra and inter-institutional transfer schemes

Prior to CATS, most health care professionals enhanced their education through non-modular 'taught courses' of a heterogeneous nature. Academic progression was in many ways tortuous with people 'progressing' from one certificate to another. For example, those who wanted to develop a career in nurse education might have followed the route described below.

First they completed their first level registration, took an English National Board course, took the Royal College of Nursing Clinical Teaching Certificate course, followed this by the University of London's Diploma in Nursing and then took the University of London's Diploma in Nursing Education to be prepared as nurse teachers with a recordable teaching qualification. All this could take at least five or six years from the point of first level registration. The point is that they still did not have a first degree and they had probably covered Maslow's hierarchy of needs on at least three occasions during previous courses!

If CAT schemes had been in operation during the early 1980s the above situation would probably have not arisen. Credit recognition and transfer would have enabled the students to move to new areas of learning without unnecessary repetition. This will be explained by referring to a typical CAT scheme.

CAT schemes incorporate a number of related concepts and terms which are important to understand. *Table 2* gives details of many of those terms as defined by the writer and may differ slightly from other published definitions.

Table 2 The 'language' of CAT schemes

Advanced standing
> the sum total of specific and general credit in relation to a particular programme of study/course

APEL
> assessment of prior experimental learning, e.g. assessment of learning related to professional practice (cf. non-certified learning)

APL
> assessment of prior learning related to award-bearing courses, e.g. degrees, diplomas and certificates (cf. certified learning)

APA
> accreditation of prior achievements (incorporating certified and non-certified learning)

Credit
> credit given for prior learning (APL and/or APEL) for which credit points are awarded:
> *general*   non-specific credit towards a programme
> *specific*   specific credit towards a programme, i.e. exemption from a particular module/modules

Credit point value
> a numerical academic value given to a module and/or prior learning at a defined level, i.e. 1, 2, 3 or M

Level
> academic level, i.e. 1, 2, 3 and M

Module
> a relatively self-contained unit of study which includes its own aims, learning processes and outcomes, content, teaching/learning strategies, scheme of assessment and indicative reading (cf credit unit; course unit)

Pathway
> a permissable route through a modular course of study leading to an educational award, e.g. degree

Professional portfolio
> a folder of evidence prepared by a student for assessment purposes

Waiver
> exemption from having to take a normally compulsory module *without being awarded credit*

The writer suggests that the philosophy of CAT schemes is based on the following values and beliefs:

• The prior experience and learning of each individual student should be highly valued and respected, consequently any APL and APEL claims should be assessed to enable relevant prior achievements and learning to be credited if appropriate.
• Students should be afforded the maximum choice in selecting modules/courses/units commensurate with their personal and professional goals.
• Students should where possible be provided with varied and flexible programmes suited to their individual needs.
• The individualized personal and academic support of every student should be a major concern of module/course unit leaders, supervisors and course co-ordinators.

Consequently, the aims of a framework for continuing professional education could be as follows:

1. To assess the prior learning/experience of every student on an individual basis.
2. To facilitate students in the identification of their learning needs.
3. To provide opportunities for students to choose an appropriate and flexible modular programme of study.
4. To provide a framework for students to achieve an appropriate academic/professional qualification.

It is important to stress that any credit that is awarded should depend on the relevance of an individual's qualifications in relation to the particular course for which the student is registered, e.g. a student with a Diploma in Management Studies is likely to be given more credit towards a BSc (Hons) in Health Services Management than towards a BSc (Hons) in Nursing Studies because of the relevance of the prior qualification to the degree in question.

The following two examples illustrate how a CAT scheme may be operated for APL claims.

APL claim – Example 1
Ward Sister RGN – Medical Ward sister
Four years post-registration experience
ENB 870 Understanding and Application of Research
City & Guilds Further Education Teaching Certificate (FETC 870)
Royal College of Nursing Certificate in Resource Management (CRM)

This student registers for a BSc (Hons) in Nursing Studies.

Advanced standing via APL =	RGN/FETC	120 points at level 1
	CRM	60 points at level 2
	ENB 870	30 points at level 2

This student would be able to claim 120 general credit points at this level 1, plus 60 general points at level 2 (CRM) and 30 specific at level 2 for a research module because of holding the ENB 870 qualification, i.e. a total of 90 credit points at level 2.

She needs 150 points including 120 at level 3 (but is not able to take any level 1 modules since no more than 120 at level 1 can be used).

Sample pathway

Year one	Credit points	Level
Compulsory nursing studies module	30	2
Optional module, e.g. a personal learning contract	20	3
Optional module, e.g. Ethics in Health Care	30	3
Year two (calendar year)		
Dissertation (compulsory)	40	3
Second compulsory nursing studies module	30	3

She is now eligible for a BSc (Hons) in Nursing Studies since she has completed all the compulsory modules and has 120 points at levels 1, 2 and 3 respectively, totalling 360 in all, the requirement for an honours degree. She may also have indexed for the English National Board's (ENB) Higher Award on entry to the degree programme.

APL claim – Example 2

Staff nurse RN (Project 2000)
6 months post-registration experience working in the community
She registers for a BSc (Hons) in Health Studies.
Advanced standing via APL: 120 credit points at level 1 & 120 at level 2
She needs 120 points at level 3.

Sample pathway

Year one	Credit points	Level
Research module (option)	20	3
Compulsory health studies module	30	3
Year two		
Optional module, e.g. Health Psychology	30	3
Dissertation (compulsory)	40	3

She is now eligible for a BSc (Hons) in Health Studies since she has completed the compulsory modules and has the 120 level 3 points to 'top up' her diploma qualification. Like the previous example, this student may also have indexed for the ENB Higher Award.

The management of APL claims is relatively straightforward provided institutions have the appropriate structures and 'tariffs of creditworthiness' for professional qualifications in relation to particular awards. It then becomes a case of looking up the value of qualifications in relation to the programme of study selected and awarding the appropriate credit points. It is acknowledged that tariffs will not be exhaustive and that *ad personam* judgements will have to be made.

The management of APEL claims is more complex, owing to the diverse nature of the claims submitted. However, if the appropriate structures and processes are in place, fair and just decisions can be made as demonstrated in the following example.

Example of an APEL claim in relation to a particular degree course

A charge nurse on part 1 of the UKCC's Professional Register wishes to register for a BSc (Hons) in Nursing Studies.

He qualified with his RGN in 1982 but did not study formally again until taking an ENB course.

He has now successfully completed the ENB 124 course Coronary Care Nursing and has produced a learning package for students allocated to his male medical ward. The purpose of the package is to provide new students with a learning resource for the care of patients following a myocardial infarction.

He is asking for a total of 120 level 1 credit points for his first level registration and ENB course and 30 general credit points at level 2 for his learning package.

He is asked to submit the following information in support of his APEL claim to the educational institution where he has applied for a degree course:

1. the learning package for assessment by two of the teaching staff.
2. a 3,000 word written assignment which includes the rationale for the package and critique.

There should also be a request for a 'letter of verification' from his clinical nurse manager regarding the learning package. It is considered very important that verification if sought for APEL claims to ensure that the work is the claimant's own, and not plagiarized.

It is very likely that the APEL claim will be endorsed providing the above three conditions have been met satisfactorily.

One of the concerns the writer has regarding CAT schemes is the way some students seem more concerned with credit than new learning. This is characterized by statements such as 'So and so will give me x amount of credit for my qualifications . . . what will you give me?' and 'Do I really have to do those modules?'

It is confusing for students because different institutions have their own interpretations of what constitutes academic level, particularly level 2 in the writer's experience. Institutions also develop and use different models for credit-rating academic/professional qualifications. One of the key quality issues for institutions of higher education is maintaining the integrity of their degree programmes while being sensitive to market forces and competitor institutions. Nevertheless, the writer remains committed to the philosophy of accreditation.

The implementation of CAT schemes nationally has been facilitated by the widespread modularization of courses. This has been essential for the philosophy of credit accumulation, recognition and transfer to be widely incorporated into the provision of continuing professional education. The principles and practice of modularization will now be explored briefly, acknowledging some of the benefits and difficulties associated with this approach to course organization and delivery.

Modularization can be described as a process of developing specific units of learning, some compulsory and some optional, which can be taken for the purpose of achieving a particular award, e.g. a certificate, diploma or degree. Some modules can also be taken on a 'stand alone' basis and may be used subsequently for credit recognition and transfer purposes.

Modularization can be conceptualized with reference to Bernstein's collection code curriculum, with strong classification and weak framing (Bernstein, 1971). He differentiates between a collection code curriculum and an integrated one. The former is characterized by strong subject boundary maintenance whereas the latter is characterized by more integration of the subject matter from different disciplines, e.g. the integration of life sciences with social and behavioural sciences.

Classification refers to the degree of insularity between curricular content or, put another way, subject separateness. Framing refers to the 'range of options available to teacher and taught in the control of what is transmitted and received in the context of the pedagogical relationship' (Bernstein, 1971 p.56).

It therefore follows that modularization in conjunction with a CAT scheme is an example of what Bernstein would call strong classification (C+) and weak framing (F–) shown in contrast to three other well-known courses for health care professionals in figure two.

Figure 2 Modularization in relation to Bernstein's Code theory

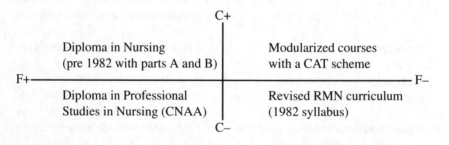

The 'old' Diploma in Nursing of the University of London was a 'taught' course with strong boundary maintenance, in part A particularly the history of learning. Individual centres may have operated a negotiated element but generally the syllabus was followed quite closely, particularly with the terminal summative examinations associated with this course. It is not the the writer's intention to criticize that particular course in this chapter (it was in fact quite hard to achieve). It has been selected as an example of strong classification and framing.

The Diploma in Professional Studies of Nursing validated by the Council for National Academic Awards (CNAA) is characterized by a more holistic approach, with more negotiation of content and delivery of this curriculum. For example, students are able to choose their own clients for en-route assignments where they are required to discuss the integrated contribution of life and social behavioural sciences to nursing care.

The delivery of the revised 1982 syllabus for part 3 of the UKCC's register has been most innovative. Students have been able to negotiate much of the content and process of their courses based on models of experiential learning.

Modularized courses based on a CAT scheme are by their nature broken down into relatively discrete units of learning (my definition in *Table 2* refers). As a corollary, the subject matter tends to have stronger boundary maintenance. The writer does not regard this as problematic since the most important consideration regarding integration is that it happens in the students' minds! For example, a student can make the links between different units of learning by using skills in transfer of learning. Secondly, the experience of producing research dissertations tends to facilitate transfer and integration of knowledge through synthesis.

Modularization associated with CAT schemes has revolutionized the structure and delivery of post-registration education in a very positive manner. Some of the main advantages and possible problems associated with this approach are suggested as follows:

Advantages	*Disadvantages*
For students	
• shorter course of study	• more demanding material at level 2/3 to learn early on in a pathway;
• acknowledgement of prior learning	• missing out on learning opportunities afforded by taking more modules; potential 'dilution' of degree studies;
• reduced cost	• cost in terms of time/money processing APEL claims;
• shared learning with other students	• missing out on culture associated with a proscribed programme of study/course;
• 'tailor-made' courses	• dilemmas over choice!
For teachers	
• job satisfaction associated with students' advantages	• time spent in advising students on advanced standing and pathway selection;
• opportunity to further develop credibility and subject expertise	• repeating teaching on modules and danger of losing enthusiasm if it is the third repeat that day!
• opportunity to work with smaller well-cohesed groups	• viability of modules with too few numbers.

For organizations

- recognition for offering a wide choice of continuing education opportunities
- increased recruitment and funding with larger student numbers
- flexible entry/transfer of students

- can be difficult to resource a number of different modules/courses
- resource intensive, e.g. need for more teachers, support services and classrooms;
- large complex schemes are very difficult to manage, e.g. a myriad of student pathways

The problems associated with managing the data generated by CAT schemes and modularization can not be overemphasised. A computerised management of information system is invaluable, if not essential, in this respect.

It has been a steep learning curve for personnel working in colleges of nursing and institutions of higher education striving to develop and sustain all the processes associated with CAT schemes and modularization. It is important that an appropriate organizational infrastructure is in place so that academic standards can be maintained. An adaptation of the Structure, Process, Outcome model described by Donabedian (1980) can be used to summarize the main principles:

Structure
It is imperative that there are formal structures to manage CAT schemes and the development of modularized courses such as Advanced Standing Committees, Module Development Panels, Programme Studies Boards and Academic Boards (different organizations will use different names within their infrastructure).
Process
The decision-making process should be equitable, based on fairness and be commensurate with academic levels.
Claims for advanced standing should be verified.
Students should have the right of appeal against awards for prior learning.
Outcomes
All decisions made by Advanced Standing Committees or their equivalent should be recorded and open to critical scrutiny. The process should be conducted with the same rigour as befits the equivalent of an examination board.
Evaluation
Evaluation should be rigorous. Data in respect of CAT schemes and modularized courses should form a major part of an institution's Quality Assurance Report.

This part of the chapter has been referred to as the 'mixed case'. It can be likened to a robust burgundy or chardonnay, rich in bouquet and flavour with a mixture of fruit and subtle undertones. CAT schemes and modularized courses are complex and can be likened to those wines. They are most welcome, full-bodied innovations in post-registration education.

In the final part of this chapter, attention will now be focused on those who provide educational experiences for both pre- and post-registration students, i.e.

teachers of nurses, midwives and health visitors (described in the remainder of this chapter as nurse teachers).

TEACHING IN A DIFFERENT WORLD

As discussed in the chapter so far, the last few years have been characterized by far-reaching and rapid change. The implementation of diploma level pre-registration courses, the shift towards total integration of Colleges of Nursing and Midwifery/Health Care Studies within Higher Education Institutions and the introduction of a market economy philosophy of educational provision, have had a significant impact on the ways in which nurse teachers function (Royal College of Nursing, 1993).

Teaching

The establishment of the Project 2000 schemes previously discussed has had a major impact on the theoretical input and the practicum of pre-registration courses. Nurse teachers now more than ever need a strong subject area knowledge, combined with intellectual and academic strength (Macleod-Clark, 1992). The potential focus of their teaching input includes:

masters degrees;	honours degrees;
P 2000 programmes;	common foundation and branches;
midwifery;	community nursing;
non-Project 2000 schemes;	continuing education;
enrolled nurse conversion;	distance learning schemes;
multidisciplinary education;	health care assistants

One of the very positive features of the qualified nurse teacher population has been the achievement of almost 100% graduate status, with many pursuing masters degrees and other higher degrees through research, i.e. masters and doctors of philosophy. In addition, all those emerging from teacher education courses are either graduates on entry or on completion.

Clinical credibility

Improving nursing education involves more than just improving the theoretical knowledge. It means achieving better clinical mastery (Rotenberg, 1986). As Gerrish (1992) postulates, nurse teachers need to develop their clinical roles to re-establish their clinical credibility, and the development of lecturer–practitioner roles has made a significant contribution in this respect. This is crucial since research has suggested that some students do not have a high opinion of teachers as role models in practice settings (Marriott, 1991).

Higher education context

Nurse teachers have also had to face a number of challenges associated with the move into higher education, including:

• different models of affiliation, e.g. working towards accredited status
• different expectations, terms and conditions of employment
• developing and maintaining academic credibility
• retaining clinical credibility
• developing research and publication skills
• developing curriculum skills
• developing organizational and administrative skills

The writer believes that this has been a salutary experience for both the nurse teacher population and their new colleagues. The development of joint appointments has facilitated a wider understanding and integration.

Market economy

The past decade has witnessed dramatic transformations in patterns of employment and unemployment in Britain (Royal College of Nursing, 1993). In nursing education, employers are making more use of temporary, short-term and part-time contracts. There has been a great deal of anxiety caused by the spectre of the three Rs, i.e. retraining, re-deployment, and redundancy, exacerbated by the Tomlinson Report (Tomlinson, 1992). It is suggested that those who remain in organizations on a full-time permanent basis will be the exceptions rather than the rule. Nevertheless, the quest for quality is paramount and in this light nurse teachers need to:

• respond to consumer/purchaser demands
• provide cost effective teaching
• monitor quality in all aspects of their work
• develop and market quality courses
• develop entrepreneurial and income-generation skills
• develop costing and budgeting skills
• develop negotiating and contracting skills
• develop political acumen

In the language of champagne, assemblage means 'the mixing of base wines to create the desired *cuvée*'. The writer proposes that nurse teachers need an 'assemblage' of the qualities and skills outlined in this section of the chapter if they are to deliver 'vintage' education. It sounds a 'tall order' but needs to be fulfilled if nurse education is to survive as a profession. It is imperative that nurse teachers respond in a positive manner to the many challenges and difficulties that lie ahead. The writer believes that they will. If they do, we can be justifiably proud of our pre- and post-registration education provision.

CONCLUSION

This chapter has covered a number of key issues germane to pre- and post-registration education. The title 'new wine in old bottles' may have led readers to suspect that the writer is doubtful as to whether the current reforms will lead to better educated nurses or whether it will be a 'case of the same old wine with new labels'! This is not the case in the writer's view, even though the prevailing economic climate affecting the country may have coloured the perception of many. As an eternal optimist, I feel that, given time and patience, the 'vintage' will be *grande marque*, i.e. high quality. As for the 'mixed case', the writer is encouraged by the developments in post-registration education. The recognition and credit for prior achievements and the modularization of undergraduate and postgraduate courses have made a national impact, opening up new doors of opportunity for thousands of nurses up and down the country. The writer is less certain about the future for nurse teachers but suggests that future preparation is likely to be characterized by mixed-mode education, combining credit for prior achievements, 'taught' modules and distance learning. In fact, such an eclectic mix may well be the norm in the delivery of education during the next quinquennium.

REFERENCES

Beattie, A. (1987) Making a curriculum work. In Allan, P. and Jolley, M. (Eds), *The curriculum in nursing education*. Croom Helm, London.

Bernstein, B. (1971) On the classification and framing of educational knowledge. In Young, M. (Ed) *Knowledge and control: new directions for the sociology of education*. Collier Macmillan, London.

Buckenham, M. (1992) Academic and organisational change. In Slevin, O. and Buckenham, M. (Eds) *Project 2000: The teachers speak*. Campion, Edinburgh.

Docking, S. (1987) Curriculum innovation. In Allan, P. and Jolley, M. (Eds) *The curriculum in nursing education*. Croom Helm, London.

Donabedian, A. (1980) *The definition of quality and approaches to its assessment*. Health Administration Press, Ann Arbor, Michigan.

ENB (1987) *Managing change in nursing education*. Pack one: *Preparing for change*. ENB: London.

Gerrish, C.A. (1992) The nurse teacher's role in the practice setting. *Nurse Education Today,* 12, 227–232.

IANE (1992) 'Assessment criteria for written work' in *Masters in Education Curriculum* document. Unpublished.

James, J. and Jones, D. (1992) Education for the future: meeting changing needs. In Slevin, O. and Buckenham, M. (Eds) *Project 2000: The teachers speak*. Campion, Edinburgh.

Jones, G.N. (1969) *Planned organisational change*. Routledge and Kegan Paul, London.

Jowett, S. (1992) Project 2000 – research on its implementation. *Nursing Times,* June 24, Volume 88, No 26 40–43.

Jowett, S., Walton, I., and Payne, S. (1991) *The NFER Project 2000 research: An introduction and some interim issues.* NFER, Slough.

Judge Report (1985) *The education of nurses: a new dispensation.* RCN: London.

Ketefian, S. (1978) Strategies of curriculum change. *International Nursing Review,* 25(1), 14–24.

Leonard, A. and Jowett, S. (1990) *Charting the course: a study of the 6 ENB pilot schemes in pre-registration nurse education.* NFER, Slough.

Marriott, A. (1991) The support, supervision and instruction of nurse learners in clinical areas. *Nurse Education Today,* 11, 261–269.

Mcleod Clark, J. (1992) *Future teachers of nurses, midwives and community nurses.* Unpublished notes from an ENB study day for the course leaders of teacher preparation courses.

Payne, S., Jowett, S. and Walton, I. (1991) *Nurse teachers in Project 2000: The experience of planning and initial implementation.* NFER, Slough.

RCN (1993) *Teaching in a different world. Report of a working party of the Education and Training Policy Committee of the Royal college of Nursing.* Unpublished.

Robinson, J.E. (1992) Mixed feelings. In *Nursing Times* September 30, Volume 88 (40) 28–30.

Rogers, E. and Shoemaker, F. (1971) *Communication of innovations: a cross cultural report,* 2nd edn. The Free Press, New York.

Rotenberg, A. (1986) Clinical teachers and teaching. *Nursing Practice* Vol 1, 203 –204.

Scrimshaw, P. (1983) *Unit 2 Educational ideologies. Educational studies: a second level course E204. Purpose and planning in the curriculum, Block 1 Society, the education system and the curriculum.* Milton Keynes: Open University.

Tomlinson, R. (1992) *Report of the Inquiry into London's Health Service, Medical Education and Research.* HMSO: London.

3.

PROCRUSTES IN THE WARD: FITTING PEOPLE INTO MODELS

INTRODUCTION

According to ancient Greek mythology, there was once a highwayman called Procrustes who lived outside Erineus in Greece. It is believed that Procrustes was not his real name. Some authors (Tripp, 1970; Comte, 1991) cite his proper name as either Damartes or Polypemon, but he was known by the nickname Procrustes, which means 'the stretcher'. He earned this nickname from the rather interesting way he treated those who came to visit his house. Comte (1991) maintains that he hijacked travellers who passed by his house on the road to Athens. Tripp (1970) cited that he invited travellers to spend the night before resuming their journey. Either way, the traveller, so the story goes, was tied to a bed in Procrustes' house. If the unfortunate traveller was too long to fit the bed, Procrustes would cut off relevant limbs until the victim did fit the bed. Conversely, if the traveller was too short for the bed, Procrustes would stretch his arms and legs so he did fit.

From this mythological tale two words or phrases have evolved. Firstly, the word 'Procrustean' now refers to the use of arbitrary or coercive methods of enforcing conformity to some kind of standard (*Encyclopedia Americana*, 1981). Secondly the phrase 'placing on Procrustes' bed' is a slang expression that refers to attempts to reduce individuals to one standard way of acting (Cooper, 1992).

So what does this mythological tale have to do with nursing?

This chapter will attempt to examine the extent to which the tale of Procrustes is analogous to the way in which nursing models are being implemented in practice. Four issues will be explored:

1. The nature of nursing theory and the relationship between theories, concepts and nursing models.
2. The application of nursing models in practice and the extent to which nursing models assist clinical decision making.
3. An exploration of two alternatives to nursing models for possible use as creative and practical tools for clinical decision making.
4. Revisiting Procrustes.

THE MEANING OF NURSING THEORY AND ITS RELATIONSHIP TO CONCEPTS AND NURSING MODELS

Within the past ten to fifteen years there has been an ever-increasing interest in developing a theory base for nursing (Field, 1987; Kristjanson *et al*, 1987; Adams, 1991; Botha, 1989). Most of this has focused on academic discourse about the nature and definition of theory. There is little evidence in the literature that is related to the application of theory to today's practice. Kristjanson *et al* (1987) expressed their concerns about the extent to which the search for a base for nursing theory will help guide the nurse in day-to-day practice. This hypothesis has yet to be proved.

Several problems arise from the increased interest in nursing theory in the literature:

1. The confusion in terminology related to theory and the inconsistency in the literature between words like theory, concept, and model.
2. If theory is an abstraction, as implied in much of the literature (Miller, 1985), questions arise as to whether it does have any relevance to the real world of nursing practice.
3. There is evidence that nurses are being pressurized (Kristjanson *et al*, 1987) explicitly or implicity to use nursing theory in practice. This may be unrealistic and leads to nurses with limited understanding of theory to attempt such application to practice.

Clarifying Terminology

Nearly all the literature related to theory development in nursing provides definitions of terminology. While there is sometimes similarity in defining terms like theory, concept, model or conceptual framework, there also is a good deal of difference in definitions (Ingram, 1991) and some evidence of misuse of terminology, which adds to nurses' confusion.

The word 'theory', for example, is defined in different ways by different writers depending upon their particular philosophical perspective. Early theoretical writers in nursing employ definitions of theory which are borrowed from the scientific community (McKay, 1969).

Botha (1989) argues that there are certain things common to all theories, in that they attempt to describe, explain, predict or control human health, illness, therapy or care, and that they provide ways of thinking about and looking at the world around us.

Chinn and Kramer (1991), on the other hand, describe theory as a set of concepts, definitions and propositions that project a systematic view of phenomena. In order to describe, predict or explain a phenomenon (in this case, nursing), theory will explain the relationship between certain concepts within that phenomenon.

Perhaps all definitions of theory can be summed up in this way: theory is an attempt to articulate what nursing is and what nurses do (or ought to do).

The purpose of nursing theory, if it is to have a practical purpose, to is explain what nurses experience in their day-to-day practice, to predict what might happen should certain actions be taken and to enable nurses to describe events. Through theory, facts are organized in a logical and cohesive way, knowledge is summarized, events predicted and the concepts that represent nursing are symbolically represented, described and explained.

Concepts are the building blocks and subject matter of nursing (Marriner-Tomey, 1989). They are mental symbols of things in the real world and could be open to many interpretations. In any theory the theorist will identify the concepts that make up the theory and will offer definitions and explanations of the concepts upon which the theory is built.

According to the literature, most theories of nursing contain certain 'key' concepts. Key concepts are the broad phenomena underpinning the theory. They are the building bricks of the theory. The concepts within a theory are joined together by suppositions or hypotheses.

Botha (1989) suggests that concepts within theories serve as mini-observation instruments which help us to organize our experiences and help us to understand our discipline.

Models of nursing are sometimes also referred to as conceptual models (Marriner-Tomey, 1989). Models are also made up of concepts. For example, Lydia Hall's model is comprised of three key concepts: behaviour, reflection and self-awareness. Peplau's model identifies and defines two major concepts: psychodynamic nursing and the nurse–patient relationship, while Orem's model of nursing identifies three key concepts: self-care, self-care deficit and nursing systems (Marriner-Tomey, 1989).

Lancaster and Lancaster (1981) suggest that theories are also models because they supposedly represent an aspect of reality. Models, however, are not theories. A model is a way of explaining something in a representational way. Models can be schematic, such as graphs, drawings or diagrams. They can also be quantitative, like mathmatical symbols. Models can also be physical, such as a model of a brain or an aeroplane. Marriner-Tomey (1989) suggests that there are two categories of models: empirical models and theoretical models. Empirical models are physical replicas of something that can be observed in the real world, like an anatomical model. Theoretical models are representations of the real world only in words or symbols. Models of nursing, therefore, are theoretical models. They are a way of symbolically putting onto paper the concepts that make up nursing, the hypotheses that bind the concepts together and the inter-relationships of the concepts with each other.

Stating our theoretical ideas about nursing is meant to help nurses understand and clarify the concepts that make up nursing before they are tested in the real world.

Models are not theories in themselves, although it is argued that they can lead to theory development (Field, 1987). Models, like theories, are made up of concepts, but models do not contain all the components that make up theory.

Lancaster and Lancaster (1981) make the point that models define and describe something, can assist in analysing something, can specify certain inter-relationships and can represent a situation symbolically. A theory, however, is more than this. Theories go beyond models by offering systematically related sets of statements, concepts or ideas which may include generalizations or propositions and which can be tested empirically.

Is there such a thing as nursing theory?

Marriner-Tomey (1989) assumes that there is such a thing as nursing theory. In doing so, she also assumes that models are representations of theories. Kristjanson *et al* (1987) present a different view. They believe that nursing is, and has been for some time, working towards developing theories. They also suggest that the majority of theoretical advances in nursing have been through the development of conceptual models (nursing models). The conceptual models that have arisen in the past ten or fifteen years are not theories in themselves because they do not provide the level of specificity required to derive principles which can be tested in practice.

Conceptual models have arisen in an attempt by nurses to define the uniqueness of nursing and these conceptual models have been in some cases inappropriately labelled as theories (Kristjanson *et al*, 1987).

For a number of reasons, the profession has put itself under a great deal of pressure to implement conceptual models into clinical practice. In doing this, with limited understanding of the model, nurses run the risk of reducing models down to individual tasks or products in much the same way as has happened with the nursing process. This reductionist approach creates systems where nurses attempt to fit their patients into the models in much the same way as Procrustes attempted to fit his victims to the bed.

THE APPLICATIONS OF MODELS IN PRACTICE AND HOW THIS INFLUENCES CLINICAL DECISION-MAKING

The use of conceptual nursing models has been dismissed by many clinical nurses. This is in part due to the way models are perceived and in the way they are presented by academics in the literature. This is compounded by the fact that the nursing process was introduced into nursing ahead of nursing models. This has resulted in the problem-solving approach of the nursing process being seen as the only legitimate approach to clinical decision-making (Henderson, 1982). The deductive approach of the nursing process, according to Henderson, largely ignored the value of intuitive judgement, which is derived from clinical knowledge and experience, not from deductive processes. This intuitive decision-making process was further elaborated by Benner (1984).

Nursing theorists may not have reached the stage where they have produced a testable theory that has all the components to enable their work to be rightly called theory.

However, in the move towards developing theory, conceptual nursing models have been identified, described and critically analysed.

The move by nursing theorists to create conceptual models was a political endeavour. The intention was not to improve nurses' ability to make clinical decisions, nor was it to improve hands-on nursing practice. Kim (1983) suggests that the achievements towards theory development through conceptual nursing models was influenced by two major considerations: it was a means to gain recognition of nursing as a profession and it was a way of providing direction for future theory development in the profession.

Ingram (1991), however, argues that all theoretical advancement in nursing should have as its purpose the improvement of nursing pratice and better patient care. If conceptual models of nursing are created solely to be tools to enhance the professional standing of nursing or for academic discourse and debate, then perhaps attempts to put them into practice as 'hands-on' tools for day-to-day nursing are inappropriate.

However, if such conceptual models are meant to enhance patient care through improving a nurse's clinical decision-making skills, then we need to move away from cavalier, recipe-book approaches to their implementation, and move towards a more considered approach for applying them in practice. This means that nurses who want to make decisions about the usefulness of a particular model need to examine the philosophical underpinnings of conceptual models and the value and belief systems upon which they are based.

All conceptual nursing models are based on certain assumptions, beliefs and values: about individuals, about the nature of health and illness, about the environment or society, and about nursing practice itself. Unfortunately, in nurses' attempt to 'do Orem' in the ward, important understandings of the philosophical underpinnings of, for example, Orem's conceptual model, have been ignored. The result seems to be that whole clinical areas are 'doing Orem' or 'using Roper' and in doing so are fitting patients into models. In short, Procrustes is alive and well in many clinical areas.

An additional observation is that the culture of nursing seems to want conceptual models to be 'finished packages' in a perfect and complete, flawless form. Yet, by very definition, conceptual models are always incomplete and always evolving. They may play a useful role in helping nurses make clinical decisions about how/what to assess in patients, but they are there to be tested and are therefore always hypothetical. Testing a model is not about 'doing' the model, it means undertaking systematic practice-based research into the validity and effects of the model and the concepts contained within it.

Field (1987) makes the point that conceptual models of nursing exist to provide nurses with tools that can be used systematically to study and examine events. One can only conclude that models are not ends in themselves but, rather, are means to ends. If this is so, what might the ends be?

The real 'end' of using conceptual models is the generation of clinical knowledge that will enhance patient care. Field (1987) cites Kuhn (1970) and Polyani (1962), who identify two types of knowledge: knowing 'that' and knowing 'how'. Nurses may know 'how' something is done without knowing 'that', e.g. the rationale for doing something.

In the case of using conceptual nursing models, a nurse may 'know that' a particular model is made up of x, y or z. What is not so easy, and therefore, less evident, is how 'knowing that' is transferred into the 'knowing how' of practice. Conceptual models of nursing, then, are tools by which nurses study their own practice, reflect on that practice, change the practice if necessary and thereby improve future practice.

Field (1987) also argues that conceptual nursing models only serve to indicate the areas of professional practice that distinguish nursing from what other health care professionals do. She also argues that models do not in themselves provide a sufficient knowledge base for making clinical judgements. This point was echoed by Benner (1984), who demonstrated that as nurses gain more experience and progress from novice to expert, they move further away from relying on their initial knowledge base to make clinical decisions.

If conceptual models of nursing form only one part of the knowledge base for nursing judgement, it is important to identify the other sources of nursing knowledge that influence the way nurses make clinical decisions.

Field (1987) identifies that another source of nursing knowledge comes from other disciplines appropriately applied to nursing. Benner (1984) argues that there is another body of nursing knowledge called practical knowledge, which is developed from experience and increased perceptual awareness and which influences clinical decision-making in experienced nurses.

Benner concluded from her research that the novice nurse operates from sets of rules when making clinical decisions. These sets of rules tend to be learned in context-free situations. For the novice, conceptual nursing models are one set of rules which she can use. Other sets of rules might be the nursing process and the procedure book. According to Benner, one characteristic of a novice is that in new or unfamiliar situations, that nurse exhibits rule-bound behaviour in narrow, limited and inflexible ways. Novices tend to apply facts, principles, conceptual models and the nursing process in rule-operated ways (Field, 1987). The recipe-book approach to using conceptual models of nursing is a characteristic of the novice nurse. It could be described as Procrustean.

The nurse who has moved to being an advanced beginner (Benner, 1984) starts to bring isolated events and situations together to form patterns that have new meaning. She can now do this as a result of having experienced, tackled, coped with and learned from enough real situations in the context of clinical settings to start noting recurring events.

The advanced beginner, however, can still be immersed in certain sets of rules to the extent that she cannot make certain important connections between pieces of information which, although they may not be obviously related to the situation at hand, may still be important to the clinical decision-making process. The advanced beginner tends to make clinical judgements from a still limited and inflexible adherence to the rules of a chosen conceptual model. However, these decisions are tempered and enriched by a small amount of context-based practical knowledge from recent experience.

The competent nurse who is using a nursing model will be one who has worked with that, or other, models for some time. Judgements related to nursing models will be conscious and will be a result of analysis of situations and problems. The competent practitioner is beginning to acquire abstract knowledge, which she uses more and more in her implementation of nursing models rather than seeking to follow the model by the letter. The competent nurse, one could argue, is also collecting data about the implementation of the model, analysing that data and beginning to examine possible refinements to the model in the face of a growing store of practical knowledge.

The proficient nurse makes judgements based on growing perceptual awareness and recent experience rather than initial factual information. Field (1987) argues that a proficient nurse who is used to using a model of nursing is more likely to be involved in seeking inter-relationships of data collected. These inter-relationships arise from a growing body of practical knowledge, and the ability to analyse data about the effectiveness of the model. This helps her relate the patient with his/her environment and with health and illness, and to make appropriate judgements for nursing actions far beyond those that are bound by the 'rules' of the model. In other words, models of nursing are adapted and changed to meet patient needs.

But it is at the expert level in nursing that the real change occurs in terms of the nurse and conceptual models of nursing. According to Field (1987) the expert nurse no longer relies on analytical principles (like the nursing process, procedural books or nursing models) to make clinical judgements and decisions. Instead, the process of making clinical judgements has become internalized. This level of perceptual awareness, according to Benner (1984), enables expert nurses to follow hunches and 'gut feelings' to make sophisticated, clinically sound judgements that bypass formal cognitive critical analysis. Similarly, Henderson (1982) referred to this process and called it the use of intuition. The expert nurse knows how to solve a problem without necessarily being able to articulate the theoretical 'knowing that'.

From this brief analysis of the development of clinical judgement skills, which takes place as the novice moves from rule-bound reliance on initial knowledge through to intuitive, sophisticated problem-solving through the development of a body of practical knowledge and perceptual awareness (expertise), it can be seen that use of nursing models in clinical practice may only be of value to the novice or advanced beginner who rely on rules for their practice and who make clinical decisions through adherence to rules.

According to Field (1987), 'nursing models give shape to the components (of nursing) and begin to define nursing and direct the goals of nursing'.

This section has attempted to examine the meaning of nursing theory and the relationships between such terms as theory, concept and model. Different perspectives have been put forward about the nature of nursing theory.

It is the author's opinion that there is little evidence that there is such a thing as 'nursing theory', and that the literature is quite conflicting about what is a nursing theory and what is a conceptual model. If there is such a group of people as nursing theorists (Marriner-Tomey, 1989) then what they have done largely is to move nursing towards possible future nursing theory, mainly through creating conceptual models. In an attempt to operationalize nursing models, the original value and belief systems underpinning them seem to have been lost. Questions have been raised about whether conceptual nursing models are only meant to be academic discussion points or whether, indeed, they have a place in enhancing patient care.

Using Benner (1984) and Field (1987), clinical application of nursing models was examined in the context of the novice to expert framework and the development of clinical judgement skills. A conclusion was drawn, which suggested that nursing models only have a place in clinical nursing as a way of providing a rule-related framework for the novice and advanced beginner, and that the competent, proficient and expert nurse develops a body of clinical knowledge and perceptual awareness or intuition that renders nursing models obsolete *vis-a-vis* clinical judgement and decision making.

The next section of this chapter will begin to examine alternatives to using nursing models as frameworks for making clinical decisions, giving care, evaluating care and ensuring high quality care.

TWO ALTERNATIVES TO CONCEPTUAL MODELS OF NURSING FOR CLINICAL DECISION-MAKING

In this section it is proposed to introduce two alternatives to the 'recipe-book' type of application of nursing models. The first alternative presents a framework from Kuypers (1986) as described by Kristjanson *et al* (1987). The framework is described by Kristjanson *et al* as a 'guiding meta-model', although Kuypers himself (1986) refers to it as 'meta-theory'.

Kuypers meta-model has been designed to enable the practitioner to examine clinical solutions and find plausible explanations for them and make choices for interventions. The meta-model is also designed to lend order to the choices made by practitioners in applying knowledge to practice and a way of enabling practitioners to articulate and discuss an infinite number of theories in practice. Hence Kuypers use of the phrase 'meta-theory' to describe this framework. It is also worth noting that Kuypers meta-theory was developed for hospital social workers. Kristjanson *et al* have attempted to apply the model to clinical decision-making in nurses.

The second alternative to using models in practice that will be offered in this section is the use of Nursing Diagnosis for clinical decision-making, giving and evaluating care and ensuring high-quality care.

Kuypers Meta-Theory for Practice

Kuypers first assumption (1986) is that all real theory occurs at the moment when the client and practitioner meet. His most fundamental, and possibly most radical, postulation is that it is the practitioner who is the theoretician. His reason for this statement is that when the practitioner first meets a client, in any setting, the practitioner is attempting from the start to understand both the unique and the common aspect of that individual situation, in other words to generate theory for and about this situation.

Applied to nursing practice, Kuypers meta-theory assumes that in the real world, practice nurses look at the data they have before them in a client situation, they look at all other available knowledge (textbook and from experience), and they also (knowingly or unknowingly) use their intuition to construct a theoretical understanding of that particular situation. In other words, the nurse is creating her own conceptual set from the real situation.

What is happening in this real patient–nurse situation provides data for the nurse which she adds to with previously gained knowledge, available theories from other disciplines and from her own intuition. This conceptual set which she creates in her own mind for this particular nursing situation serves a number of functions.

Firstly, it provides some kind of direction to the nurse's enquiries about the patient. Secondly, it enables the nurse to organize her observations of the patient into patterns which facilitate the identification of their health concerns. Thirdly, it enables appropriate clinical decisions to be made, which can be articulated and which have a theoretical and practical knowledge-based rationale.

Kuypers meta-theory applied to nursing is based on three domains or constructs: the domain of health, the domain of error, and the domain of change. The nurse can create theoretical statements or practical theory about each of these three domains for each patient situation. Kuypers believes that this is done by addressing each client situation using a simple process of scientific enquiry. This involves the nurse asking three questions (adapted from Kuypers, 1986):

1. What is the health state that this person wishes to have (ideal)?
2. What error is preventing this ideal from happening?
3. What change should occur to enable this client to achieve the health state he or she wishes?

These questions, as a process of scientific enquiry, enable the nurse to become the practical theoretician. In order to understand the questions within the process of scientific enquiry, it may be helpful to examine the three domains in greater depth.

The Domain of Health

In this domain the nurse and client work together to enable the nurse to create a theory for the health of this client. To do this the nurse engages in a sort of scientific enquiry process related to health and, in the attempt to create such a theory, asks the first of the three questions (above). The nurse will gather data from and about the client related to health and the two will come to some sort of decision as to what constitutes optimum health for this client.

This definition of health may range from an ideal view of optimum health in terms of maximum human potential (Kristjanson *et al* 1987) or a more practical statement of immediate short-term health goals. The nurse will be influenced by formal theoretical definitions, for example, models of health. The end result is that a practical theory of health for this client's unique situation is created, which then forms the basis for nursing decisions, goal setting and interactions.

The Domain of Error

In this domain the nurse attempts to construct a theory about the forces or circumstances that may account for what is happening to the client/patient now, and why it is falling short of the optimum health desired for the patient. The practical theory the nurse is seeking to create is an answer to the question, 'how is it the desired healthy state doesn't exist?' In creating a theory for this client's actual situation, the nurse is seeking possible explanations for the source of this error. The explanations uncovered will have an impact on the clinical decisions the nurse makes about nursing interventions.

The Domain of Change

This third domain requires the nurse to construct a theory for the client in this situation about what sort of change might be required in order to enable the client to achieve his/her desired health state. Here, the nurse will rely on an understanding of change theories that will influence the clinical judgements and decisions made.

The three domains enable the nurse to create theory from real clinical situations, which then guides clinical decisions about the patient. It is a fundamental move away from 'grand theory', which attempts to explain all nursing situations from one theoretical perspective. Instead, Kuypers approach calls for the nurse to be her own theoretician by generating theory, from each client situation, which is relevant and appropriate for the clinical judgements required for that particular client.

Kuypers makes overt the reality that theory exists to help nurses make clinical judgements. However, rather than choosing a particular theory, or group of theories as the starting point for the clinical decision made, Kuyper's model invites the nurse to begin with the reality of a patient–nurse situation and then to generate practical theory from that situation. This practical theory will be unique to the patient's needs and will be created by the nurse through a structured enquiry process, using presenting data from and about the patient, available theories from the literature as appropriate, knowledge (textbook and experiential) and intuition. This in turn influences clinical judgement and decision making to find the best solutions for that particular client in that particular situation.

The process, however, is influenced by other things, namely, by how the nurse herself deals with uncertainty, and her awareness that there is no one correct answer (Kristjanson *et al*, 1987). In addition, her own value and belief system will also influence interpretation of data (Botha, 1989). The meta-model, however, takes account of this whereas using another person's conceptual model may not.

By using Kuypers' meta-model, nurses begin to generate theory from the real-life work situation, which, although it can be 'fraught with tension and doubt' (Kuypers 1986) in the decision making process, enables the nurse to realize, upon reflection, that the choices made are unique and specific to this client situation. Kuyper also speculates that nursing's recent history of trying to use grand theory to make decisions is an attempt to make decision-making more comfortable.

Using Kuypers' meta-theory approach as an alternative to taking an existing conceptual model and applying it to practice raises a number of issues:

1. The meta-theory approach described by Kuypers (1986) requires a high degree of personal professional accountability. The nurse does not use a named conceptual model as justification for clinical decisions. Instead she justifies clinical decisions from her own theory for that patient in that situation. Therefore, the nurse needs to demonstrate that she can articulate the process behind the clinical decision.
2. Clinical judgement is open to scrutiny.
3. Using the meta-theory approach provides the potential for increased choices in clinical decision making but, according to Kuypers (1986), if choices are made without awareness, then the range of options decreases and the possibility of uncritical ritual and rigidity increases.
4. Generating theory specific to each patient using this meta-theory approach requires the nurse to have moved away from practice that is rule-governed, as in Benner's description of the novice and advanced beginner (1984). Therefore, to use meta-theory will require the development of perceptual awareness (Benner 1984), clinical knowledge and experience, which will lead to proficient and expert practice.

Nursing Diagnosis

The second alternative to using conceptual models in practice is the use of nursing diagnosis. The idea of nursing diagnosis was first suggested in the 1950s, but it was only in the 1970s that American nurses began to seriously identify nursing diagnosis as a way of distinguishing the profession of nursing from the medical profession. In this respect it has followed a similar political history to conceptual models in nursing. Although the concept of a nursing diagnosis was first identified as a stage in the nursing process that came after data collection and before problem identification (planning), nursing diagnoses now are seen to have the potential for guiding clinical decision-making in its own right.

As a clinical decision-making tool, nursing diagnoses have some similarity to Kuypers meta-theory framework. Both of them rely on data collection from real nursing situations and making clinical judgements about the relationships within that data. Both of them require the nurse to combine this observational data with previous textbook knowledge, other theory and practical knowledge. A nursing diagnosis is a way of assigning a name to a group of signs, symptoms and other observational data which is of concern to nurses and nursing.

Giving a name (a nursing diagnosis) to this collection of signs, symptoms and other data enables nurses to have a common language which they can use to communicate with each other, and which has shared meaning and understanding.

Ziegler et al (1986) call nursing diagnoses 'first level theory development'. It is an attempt to generate theory from real experience and in this respect shares similar aims with Kuypers' meta-theory. Ziegler et al (1986) explain that developing a nursing diagnosis is a process in itself. This process is made up of determining cues by examining the data collected from a patient and comparing this to norms and standards suggested by the literature and from research. This may include using theories from other disciplines as a part of that literature. This is the first part of the process of making a nursing diagnosis. The next stage in the process is where the nurse combines clusters of cues (from observing and assessing a patient) into groups or patterns. In doing so the nurse creates clearly articulated labels for these patterns. These in turn are checked against the literature, research and the nurse's store of practical knowledge.

The process continues with the nurse drawing conclusions about any unhealthful patterns (Field, 1987) and creating an aetiology or name for these unhealthful patterns. This aetiology or name is the nursing diagnosis. There are now published texts that classify and list nursing diagnoses that have been nationally agreed in the United States, e.g. Hurley, 1986.

Two problems appear to have arisen from the nursing-diagnosis approach to clinical decision-making. One is the word 'diagnosis', which many nurses find unacceptable because of its medical connotation. The second problem, identified by Field (1987), is that nursing diagnoses direct none of their focus on the patient's strengths or on the factors that might have led to or influenced the severity of the nursing diagnosis. This, according to Field, is a particular problem when using nursing diagnoses in community nursing settings.

Data collection from patients is not a new part of nursing practice. Field (1987), however, found that nurses were able to collect data but that they were unable to critically examine that data and identify relationships between pieces of information. As a result, their clinical judgements were poor and they did not necessarily arrive at appropriate conclusions.

Using nursing diagnoses to make clinical judgements is not reliant on any particular conceptual nursing model. Data comes from the real nursing situation and is supplemented by literature, research and practical knowledge. It is a way in which steps towards theory development (Ziegler *et al*, 1986) can take place from practice.

Field (1987) also makes a plea for nurses to realise that, although nursing diagnoses are independent from medical diagnoses, they should not be considered in isolation from each other. Medical diagnoses can be used in two ways as part of the process of making a nursing diagnosis.

Firstly, medical diagnoses can be re-interpreted into a nursing perspective and secondly, this re-interpretation of medical diagnoses becomes part of the literature/theory from other disciplines, which is then applied to nursing.

Summary of the Alternatives to Conceptual Models

Both Kuypers' meta-theory (1986) and nursing diagnoses offer alternative approaches to conceptual nursing methods as practical tools for clinical decision-making. Both alternatives present a practice-based approach to theory development which promotes the notion of the nurse as practical theoretician. Both alternatives attempt to demonstrate ways in which theory generation begins with real patient data which is supplemented by existing literature and clinical knowledge and research. Kuypers' meta-theory offers the added dimension of the use of intuition in this process, a view supported by Benner's notion of perceptual awareness influencing clinical decision-making.

PROCRUSTES REVISITED

This account began with the tale of Procrustes, and has attempted to show how conceptual models of nursing have, metaphorically, led nurses to act like Procrustes with their patients. Through lack of understanding of the purpose of conceptual models, all too often patients have been made to fit the models in rule-bound application of such models to practice. Three conclusions can be tentatively drawn from the arguments and discussions within this chapter:

1. Conceptual models of nursing may be appropriate tools to aid clinical judgement and decision-making for novices and advanced beginners in nursing because of their rule-bound reliance upon decision-making
2. Alternatives to conceptual nursing models, such as the two suggested in this chapter, might be more appropriate frameworks for clinical decision-making in proficient and expert nurses
3. Nurses' approaches to the use of conceptual models in practice and the extent to which they seek alternatives to such models to guide clinical decision-making may be an indicator of their own development along the novice-to-expert continuum.

Perhaps the vision of the future for the expert nurse might herald a re-writing of the story of Procrustes as follows:

'Procrustes was a highwayman in Greece who lived in a house by the side of the main road between Erineus and Athens. He used to invite travellers to spend the night in his house before continuing their journeys. If the traveller was too big or too small for the bed, Procrustes would cut the bed to size or make it bigger to enable the traveller to fit into it more comfortably'.

REFERENCES

Adams, T. (1991) The idea of revolution in the development of nursing theory. *Journal of Advanced Nursing*, 16(12), 1387–1491.

Benner, P. (1984) *From Novice to Expert*. Addison–Wesley, Menlo Park.

Botha, M.E. (1989) Theory development in perspective: the role of conceptual frameworks and models in theory development. *Journal of Advanced Nursing*, 14(1), 49–55.

Chinn, P. and Kramer, M. (1991) *Theory and Nursing: a Systematic Approach*, 3rd edn. Mosby, St. Louis.

Comte, F. (1991) *Mythology*. Chambers, Edinburgh.

Cooper, J.F. (1992) *Brewer's Myths and Legends*. Cassell, London.

Fawcett, J. (1980) A framework for analysis and evaluation of conceptual models of nursing. *Nurse Educator*, 5(6), 10–4.

Field, P.A. (1983) An ethnography: four public health nurses' perspectives of nursing. *Journal of Advanced Nursing*, 8(1), 3–12.

Field, P.A. (1987) The impact of nursing theory on the clinical decision-making process. *Journal of Advanced Nursing*, 12(5), 563–71.

Henderson, V. (1982 The nursing process – is the title right? *Journal of Advanced Nursing*, 7(2), 103–9.

Hurley, M. (Ed) (1986) *Classification of Nursing Diagnoses: Proceedings of the Sixth Conference*. Mosby, St. Louis.

Ingram, R. (1991). Why does nursing need theory? *Journal of Advanced Nursing*, 16(3), 350–3.

Kim, H.S. (1983) *The Nature of Theoretical Thinking in Nursing*. Appleton–Century–Crofts, Norwalk.

Encyclopedia Americana, Vol 22 (1981). Grolier, Danbury.

Kristjanson, L.J., Tamblyn, R. A model to guide development and application of multiple nursing theories. *Journal of Advanced Nursing*, 12(4), 523–9.

Kuhn, T. (1970) *The Structure of Scientific Revolution*, 2nd edn. University of Chicago Press, Chicago.

Kuypers, J.A. (1986) *The H-E-C framework: examining theory choices in clinical social work*. Unpublished paper, School of Social Work, University of Manitoba.

Lancaster, W. and Lancaster, J. (1981) Models and model building in nursing. *Advances in Nursing Science*, 3(3), 31–42.

McKay, R. (1969) Theories, models and systems for nursing. *Nursing Research*, 18(5), 393–400.

Marks-Maran, D. (1992). Rethinking the nursing process. In *Nursing Care: The Challenge to Change*, Jolley, M. and Brykczynska, G. (Eds), pp.91–10. Edward Arnold, London.

Marriner-Tomey, A. (1989). *Nursing Theorists and Their Work*, 2nd edn. Mosby, St. Louis.

Miller, A. (1985) The relationship between nursing theory and nursing practice. *Journal of Advanced Nursing*, 10(5), 417–24.

Polyani, M. (1962) *Personal Knowledge*. Routledge and Kegan Paul, London.

Tripp, E. (1970) *Cromwell's Handbook of Classical Mythology*. Cromwell, New York.

Ziegler, S.M., Vaughan-Wrobel, B.C. and Erlen, J.A. *Nursing Process, Nursing Diagnosis, Nursing Knowledge: Avenues to Autonomy*. Appleton–Century–Crofts, Norwalk.

4.

ADDRESSING THE CHALLENGE OF THE THEORY/PRACTICE GAP

PART ONE: THE THEORY–PRACTICE GAP REVISITED

An ongoing debate in the development of nursing as a discipline is that of the relationship between theory and its practice. The literature seldom portrays it as an easy or straightforward issue, even less as one that has been resolved (Miller, 1985; Speedy, 1989). Before looking at the contribution of the developing role of lecturer practitioner to this debate, it is useful to examine once again the disparity that is said to exist between theory and practice. In this way the possibilities of the lecturer practitioner's role can be demonstrated in relation to the apparent dichotomy between the practice and theory of nursing. The nature, antecedents and results of the so-called theory–practice gap are briefly considered here. This will be followed by an examination of the lecturer practitioner role in terms of the conditions required and the potential contributions of the role to bringing theory and practice together in nursing practice, education, management and research.

Aspects of Theory

A view that persists in nursing is that of theory being a separate entity from the practice of nursing: 'Nursing has had a historical tendency toward polarization dichotomies.' (Meleis, 1985)

The position of theory and practice as polar opposites seems to be accepted as fact with little thought as to the properties of theory and practice themselves. Jarvis (1992) points out that discussion about the relationship between theory and practice is problematic since neither term is clearly defined. It is suggested here that an examination of theory and practice demonstrates a complexity that may provide us with clues as to how they may be reconciled and how it may be possible, even desirable, to live with an apparent paradox (Meleis, 1987).

Theory is not a single entity. Pearson (1989) has suggested that it takes various forms; theories personal to an individual, local theory, grand theory, and so on. People produce theory in different ways and at different levels. Nursing has traditionally accorded most credibility to theory drawn from the natural and physical sciences. Such theory is characterized by its emphasis on control, measurement, reductionism and objectivity (Allen, 1985; Hagell, 1989). Arguably the influence of such a prevailing paradigm has manifested itself in hierarchial and compartmentalized work roles which, to an extent, still persist. However, such assumptions are at odds with contemporary nursing thought. Traditional conceptions of scientific rigour are being seen as inadequate in addressing broad human issues (Tilden and Tilden, 1985). With the espousal of a more holistic view of nursing's clients comes the pursuit of an understanding that also encompasses emotion and subjectivity (Pearson, 1989).

For nurses, theory can mean different things. For the students in Melia's (1987) study (and one suspects, for many nurses past and present) theory was what was found in books, taught in the school of nursing, or the medical background to 'basic' nursing care. Such theory can be seen as having only limited value for practising nurses caring for patients inasmuch as it has been characterized as lacking rationale and scope.

Until relatively recently, the theory taught in schools of nursing has been derived largely from medicine. Even where it has been produced by nurses, the care prescribed has been built around a medical model. More recently, other sources of theory have been employed deductively in the education of nurses, especially within centres of further education; psychology, sociology, education, microbiology, and so on. Champion (1983) has pointed out that this eclecticism has added further complexity to the nature of theory utilized in nursing. The various disciplines have differing bodies of knowledge. They also employ methodologies fundamental to the understanding of their theoretical content.

As a result, the development of nursing knowledge has been contributed to by various groups subscribing to quite distinct paradigmatic positions, that is to say, particular ways of seeing and interpreting the world (Kuhn, 1970). Champion suggests that teachers of one discipline usually have little appreciation of the methods or content of subjects other than their own. Moreover, rival approaches within disciplines develop; for instance, quantitative versus qualitative research methods in the various social sciences.

Apart from the various bodies of knowledge used deductively by nursing, there is the fast growing body of nursing theory itself. The exact nature, purpose and utility of nursing theory is a matter of continuing debate. Controversy in itself is no bad thing (Pearson, 1989). Without discussion, new and refined answers cannot be arrived at. Nonetheless, for practising nurses exhorted to adopt the nursing process, nursing models, primary nursing, and so on, the situation can become very confusing.

Theory Guiding Practice

Fawcett (1980) wrote: 'The purpose of theory is to explain relevant events in the world, and in a practice discipline . . . to provide knowledge which can be used as a guide to direct the actions of members of that discipline.'

This is a view attributed to those nursing scholars seeking to mould nursing in the shape of a scientific tradition (e.g. Beckstrand, 1978). In it the relationship between theory and practice is seen as essentially one way. Researchers and theorists build the theories that practitioners in turn use to guide their practice. One manifestation of this approach is the nursing model (Speedy, 1989).

Some nursing models are said to be derived inductively, that is to say, derived from the practice of nursing (e.g. Roper *et al*, 1983). The majority are derived deductively from more or less arcane social and scientific theory (Roy, 1984; Rogers, 1980; Parse, 1981; Patterson and Zderad, 1986). The debates between the various disciples of the different models add yet more layers to the complexity of nursing theory.

Even supposing that the various models of nursing have something to offer to nursing practice, and there exists no conclusive proof that they do (Chapman, 1990), recent experience has thrown up a number of barriers between the idealization and practice of nursing. For example, models have been adopted uncritically, instead of as a tool to be adapted critically by the user (Gordon, 1984; Lister, 1987). As a result there may have been little more than a swapping of one set of rules for another (Hardy, 1982). Some research has suggested that, for practising nurses, the adoption of nursing models has proved restrictive rather than facilitative to practice (Gordon, 1984; Price, 1987). A further, frequently cited barrier to the use of models is their difficult language (Gordon, 1984; Gruending, 1985; Miller, 1985). The major source of nursing models is the USA. Nurses using these models in the UK have discovered that such models are in some ways culturally inappropriate to practice in the National Health Service (NHS) (Wright, 1986; Draper, 1990).

It could be argued that fundamental to this catalogue of problems is the fact that the models are not adequately shaped by practice (Benner and Wrubel, 1989). Models have been used more to shape educational curricula than practice itself, so creating dissonance for nurses in training, who are confronted by a world of practice that differs from that they have learnt. This is not, however, a problem unique to current nursing theory. The nursing procedures and tasks that were taught in schools of nursing traditionally seldom matched the realities of practice (Bendall, 1975).

Fawcett (1980) stresses the role of research in the guidance of practice by theory. She writes that theory frames the research questions that in turn refine the theory. However, to date, the relationship between research and practice has not been straightforward. Over the last thirty years in the UK and longer in the USA, nursing has been subject to an increasing amount of research both by nurses and by those interested in nursing. However, an issue that is frequently raised is why the knowledge derived from research so rarely has an impact on practice (Hunt J., 1981, 1984; Hockey, 1983; Greenwood, 1984; Hunt M., 1987). Various possible reasons as to why this is have been advanced, such as:

• the availability of findings
• the comprehensibility of findings
• nurses do not have the authority to use findings
• nurses do not know how to use findings

Greenwood (1984) suggests that research findings are not used because many research studies do not focus on issues that are relevant to practising nurses. MacGuire (1990) argues that in terms of what is now known about the complexity of the process of change the arguments of earlier commentators may have been premature. Change, she says, is more than a rational response to the demonstration of factual information. For example, Hunt (1988), writing about the popularity of primary nursing, observed that research evidence has little to do with decisions to change if an idea appeals strongly to those who want it to happen!

The stance that the relationship between theory and practice is one of theory guiding practice can, then, be questioned: '. . . nursing care requires more than science for its legitimacy and direction.' (Benner and Wrubel, 1989, p.20)

The purpose of the positivist scientific paradigm can be said to be the discovery of universal, context-free laws that account for irregularities and patterns in the world. Laws describe cause-and-effect relationships that explain what is happening and predict outcomes. The goal of this way of seeing the world can be said to be achieved through explaining and predicting events (Hagell, 1989). Such a position has proved to be unsatisfactory in providing an adequate basis for nursing practice, just as it has for other groups such as social workers and teachers. It has already been noted that there are many ways of developing and describing theory. Recently there has been a growing trend to acknowledge and develop the theoretical knowledge embedded in the practice of nurses.

Practice Guiding Theory

Clarke (1986) wrote: '. . . practical activity is primary but . . . theoretical activity arises from practice and serves to modify it.'

This point of view is also represented in the work of Benner (1984), amongst others. Those who hold this view suggest that theory to guide practice is embedded within practice itself. Both theory and practice are as important as each other, as theory frames the issues and guides the practitioner in where to look and what to ask. But, argue Benner and Wrubel (1989), expert practice can go beyond the current state of learning and so further enrich theory. Clinical situations are always more varied and complicated than theoretical accounts, and therefore clinical practice is an arena of inquiry and knowledge development. For, as Carr and Kemmis (1986) have said, practice is not carried out in isolation from theorizing. The practitioner is guided by some sort of theory in their practice.

In practical terms this means exploring new ways of uncovering nursing knowledge. For researchers, this has lead to the use of various qualitative research approaches such as phenomenology, ethnography, grounded theory, and so on (cf. Leininger, 1985; Munhall and Oiler, 1986), which emphasize the participation, to a greater or lesser degree, of the research informants. Other strategies to improve the relevance of research and theorizing to practice include the development of action research methodologies that directly involve practitioners in identifying problems and attempting to solve them (Lathlean, 1989; Webb, 1989). Indeed, such work need not be done by an outside researcher but by the informants themselves (FitzGerald, 1989). Various other collaborative projects have also been described (Wilson-Barnett et al, 1990). Although their value has yet to be formally evaluated, it could be argued that what is striking about this work is its apparent relevance to the area studied.

Practising nurses also need to learn how to recognize and develop the knowledge that they use in their practice. Influential in this have been the works of Schon (1987) and Smyth (1986) amongst others. Schon, writing about architectural practice, stresses the importance of moving away from the 'high, hard ground' of manageable problems to the 'swampy lowlands' of the complex and imperfect world of practice. Practitioners need to develop skills of reflecting critically on the impact of their practice. Practice may then perhaps be used to challenge and refine theory by validating it within a practice setting (Chinn and Jacobs, 1983). Moreover, attention must be paid to the authority and autonomy of practising nurses if they are to be able to both collectively and individually evolve their practice.

Carr and Kemmis (1986), two educationalists, have written about the notion of 'praxis'. Praxis is a term used to describe the reasoning for action. Praxis is constructed through action and by reflecting on the process and outcomes of actions compared with the reasons and intentions of the action in a given situation. Such reflection-in-action (Schon, 1987) is said to advance and develop the knowledge base of a practitioner. Carr and Kemmis (1986) take the idea still further. Through praxis, a practitioner can reconcile the supposedly opposed notions of theory and practice. For this to occur a practitioner is required who can rationally apply theory to decision making with consideration of the context, reflecting critically on the action and its consequences in order to construct new thought relevant to the situation.

Given the highly diverse nature of the growth, development and use of theory in nursing, it is difficult to come to a firm conclusion about a current 'state of the art'. The trend in nursing seems to be moving away from the evolution and promotion of broad, 'grand' theory, such as that contained in nursing models, to an acknowledgement of the importance of theory that is more specific in nature and that evolves in response to the experience of practice.

Aspects of Nursing Practice

Practice is no more a single entity than theory is. Practitioners themselves vary as individuals, and between clinical and geographical areas. Motivation differs, preparation differs, expectations differ. As a crude example, at teaching hospitals young people with good exam results prepare for a career, while in small district hospitals married women with children choose between a limited number of options and choose to work at what is often the largest source of women's employment in the area (Clarke, 1978).

The variation within clinical nursing has been demonstrated in a number of research studies. Schröck (1973) found that a ward's label was no reliable guide to the educational experience to be gained there. Studies by Fretwell (1982), Orton (1981) and Ogier (1982) suggested that the learning climates on different wards differed according to, amongst other things, characteristics of organization and leadership, and that a vital factor was the role taken by the ward sister or nurse in charge.

Nursing practice, until relatively recently, has arguably been the poor relation of the four pillars of nursing (practice, education, management and research), even though it is the *raison d'etre* for the whole nursing profession. This status is reflected in ward hierarchies where nursing work is differentiated according to ideas of seniority – students bath the patients, staff nurses answer phones, sisters do the ward rounds, etc (Melia, 1987). In some areas this is changing, but not in all. To pursue a career in nursing it is necessary to move away from practice, performing 'lateral arabesques' (Kramer, 1974) into the arenas of education, management or research. By and large this transition is only possible by gaining further qualifications. The transition usually carries with it status, regular hours and a higher salary. The clinical regrading exercise of 1988 has done a little to address this problem. Nonetheless, the career structure of nursing in the UK encourages nurses away from the bedside, and does little to encourage them to return. It is from the cohorts of those who have left practice for management, education and research that the exhortations to change most often come. However, this 'top down' approach to bringing about change is increasingly being seen as less effective than a 'bottom up' approach, which directly involves those expected to change (Wright, 1989).

Preparation for Practice

The preparation of new practitioners has traditionally been in the hands of those who have to a greater or lesser extent left practice behind them. Research and enquiries into the plight of student nurses as they journey between the school of nursing and the wards have highlighted a number of problems: a state of tension between the learning needs of students, the aspirations of the school of nursing and the staffing needs of the nursing service (Committee on Nursing, 1972; Bendall, 1975); a low degree of relevance and integration between taught material and the experience of students in practice (Alexander, 1983; Melia, 1987), a conflict for which students were not entirely prepared (Gott, 1984). Various methods of resolving these problems have been addressed, such as examining the educational role of sisters/charge nurses and creating the post of clinical teacher, each with limited success.

The teaching of student nurses is frequently included in the job description of senior nurses, ward sisters and charge nurses. Yet evidence suggests that it is not always a priority (Fretwell, 1982), neither are its particular demands accounted for in calculating workload (Vaughan, 1989). The preparation of sisters for their teaching role is not always adequate (Farnish, 1983). As early as the 1950s it became clear that the responsibility for the teaching of practice could no longer be vested in the ward sister alone. Nonetheless, as will be illustrated, the need for the leader of a nursing team to be central in establishing both learning climate and professional socialization in a clinical area has been preserved and redefined within the remit of the lecturer practitioner.

The role of clinical teacher came into being as a means of helping students to integrate theory and practice and to supervise their clinical work (Lathlean, 1990). However a number of problems became apparent within the role. The clinical teacher was a visitor to a ward and had no formal authority or responsibility for the clinical area in which she/he was supposed to teach practice. The clinical teacher's credibility was compromised by the lack of continuity in her/his work, since they were not on wards for any period of time. There existed also the possibility of losing credibility in the eyes of students and ward nurses through not working within the constraints of the reality of practice; for example, the teacher and student looking after a small caseload of patients. While this may be understandable in that the teacher's prime responsibility is helping students learn, it does not necessarily help the students face the reality of the work situation (Vaughan, 1990).

A large scale survey of nurse educators undertaken by the General Nursing Council (1975) identified the following as the cause of greatest dissatisfaction amongst clinical teachers: inadequate recognition of their job; inadequately delineated areas of responsibility; and the conflict between education and service. Clinical teachers as a separate grade were not generally accepted either as educators or as clinical nurses (Wright, 1981, cited in Lathlean, 1990). Partly as a result of such problems and with the advent of Project 2000, clinical teachers are now being phased out.

There is then a problem of views of nursing theory being separate from views of nursing practice. It is not difficult to understand why such a gap is thought to exist. However, it could be argued that the gap in fact exists between a certain kind of theory and a certain way of seeing practice, that is to say, theory which is for various reasons irrelevant to practice, and a view of practice which sees it as inferior to theory rather than a spring from which theory for nursing practice can evolve.

Both theory and practice have been presented here as complex and diverse notions. Theory in nursing has historically been informed by contrasting scientific traditions. There is a body of thought to suggest that the theoretical positions derived from other disciplines are not adequate to describe or guide nursing. Consequently, there is now a movement towards discovering and developing the theory embedded in nursing practice. It can be argued that, for this to happen, nurses should be better equipped to analyse and develop their own practice. However, it has also been suggested here that the preparation of new practitioners is problematic in a variety of ways. As a result, the search continues for a means by which the efforts of nursing education and nursing practice can become more congruent.

PART TWO: LECTURER PRACTITIONERS – A NEW RESPONSIBILITY FOR PRACTICE

There is a challenge to create a practice environment in which theory and practice can inform each other. From the mid-1980s work began within Oxfordshire Health Authority on a range of measures aimed towards the provision of quality professional nursing practice, the basic premise being that all patients have the right to be nursed by qualified nurses who are knowledgeable, skillful and capable of making nursing decisions without deferring to higher authority (FitzGerald, 1989).

Reports on problems in the recruitment and retention of learners have highlighted a variety of problems, including the apprenticeship style of training, learners' inclusion in service establishments (Committee on Nursing, 1972), the high proportion of non-nursing work and the cursory attention paid to education (Fretwell, 1982). Early plans for the development of nursing in Oxford were oriented to addressing these problems through the re-evaluation of the whole nursing service.

Commitment to continuing education was increased through the formation of a clinical practice development team. Post-basic education was actively encouraged and nursing development was carried out in a variety of areas, for example, the Burford and Oxford Nursing Development Units (Pearson, 1983; 1989). The subsequent undergraduate programme was planned bearing in mind the nursing developments within the district. The purpose of the course is: 'The preparation of academically able people with a desire to pursue a career in clinical nursing . . . as professional practitioners of nursing.' (Oxford Polytechnic Vol. 1, p.52)

The notion of nursing being a practice-led profession (Ryan, 1989) resulted in the course-planning teams being heavily influenced by educationalists such as Schon, Argyris, Boud and Keough, who emphasize the importance of the real world of practice as a source of learning for practitioners, and by nursing theorists such as Benner, who examined the process through which nurses develop expertise (Champion, 1988). A common factor in the work of the above is their acknowledgement of the complexity and contextually dependent nature of professional practice.

Providing professional nursing practice

A central problem in providing professional nursing is that, while the authority for the teaching and practice of nursing are vested in different groups of people, the dissonance created by the discrepancies between what is done and what is taught will remain. Indeed, as nursing's body of knowledge grows and nursing education is moved to centres of higher education (a prominent feature of some of the Project 2000 curricula that are currently being implemented) the perceived theory–practice gap may well increase. Moreover, it is unlikely that the practice of clinical nursing will be developed as effectively while such discrepancies remain (Vaughan, 1990).

Historically, various attempts have been made to address the problem. Through the the analysis of change in social policy proposed by Vickers (1983, cited in Vaughan, 1989) Vaughan has argued that a new approach to nursing structure is required.

Vickers suggests that when a particular role is seen to be ineffective, a first approach is to split off part of that role; for example, the introduction of the clinical teacher, which was intended to complement and support the ward sister's educative role. With this partition comes the problems of split authority. The clinical teacher had no formal authority to change practice even if it was incongruent with what she/he was teaching.

A second approach is to add responsibilities to a role. Vaughan (1989) likens this to the development of joint appointees. The notion of joint appointments was suggested as a means of bridging the gap between education and service (Committee on Nursing, 1972). Wright (1983) outlined the following themes as comprising the role of the joint appointee:

- As a teacher in the classroom and on the wards, teaching nursing, management and research
- Synthesizing the roles of trained teacher and experienced nurse in charge of care provision
- As manager of a clinical area
- As a developer of research into nursing

Joint appointment posts proved highly demanding and although there were many positive aspects to the arrangement, various studies describe a situation where those holding the posts 'became separately identified in the minds of the staff within the school and the service area.' (Balogh and Bond, 1984). Instead of being a unifying force they were seen as different from both nurses and nurse–teachers. Vaughan (1989) suggests that it was a case of two roles being combined with little thought as to what could be discarded or delegated.

Vickers (1983) cited by Vaughan 1989 describes a third approach. That is, to look for a fundamental change, dismantling what is in existence and restructuring it entirely. It is with this approach in mind that the role of lecturer practitioner has been developed.

The role of the lecturer practitioner

'The lecturer practitioner is a senior nurse who has a mastery of practice, education, management and research. Through demonstrating these collective skills s/he (*sic*) is able to lead a team of nurses delivering a professional service to patients, at the same time developing personal skills and knowledge in her/himself and the nurses working alongside.' (FitzGerald, 1989, p.13).

The discussion of the role of the lecturer practitioner is based on how it has been defined and developed within Oxfordshire Health Authority. The title is now used in several parts of the country and while it is a new and developing role, there will inevitably be differences in its various applications. In Oxford, lecturer practitioners have responsibility and authority for both practice and education within a defined clinical area. They are directly accountable to the director of nursing services and the head of the Department of Health Care Studies at Oxford Brook University. Vaughan (1990) delineates two chief areas of responsibility:

1. To identify and maintain the standards of practice and policies within a defined clinical area.
2. To prepare and contribute to the educational programme of students in relation to the theory and practice of nursing in that unit.

   Not all lecturer practitioners within the Health Authority are the same. Lathlean (1990) describes four models:

• Lecturer practitioner, ward manager (sister role) and unit manager (senior sister role)
• Lecturer practitioner and ward manager
• Lecturer practitioner and unit manager
• Lecturer practitioner alone, working collegially with a ward sister

   This discussion is based around the implications of the first model. In order to control the clinical environment for both patient care and student learning, the lecturer practitioner's managerial responsibilities include:

• developing ward philosophies, goals and frameworks for practice in conjunction with the rest of the clinical team
• acting as a clinical consultant to the ward/unit team
• having a clinical role (intermittently or continuously as dictated by other demands of the role), either through having a clinical caseload or acting as an associate nurse
• monitoring the quality of nursing and feeding back to the ward team and hospital management
• developing nurses' contribution within the multidisciplinary team, as well as developing communication networks within the unit, in the district and nationally
• facilitating research-based practice and clinical research on the ward
• managing the nursing budget, developing the skill mix and appointing new staff (FitzGerald, 1989; Vaughan, 1990).

   The Griffiths report (NHS Management Inquiry Team, 1983) had lent support to the development of a nursing structure intended to flatten the hierarchy and facilitate professional practice. Senior sisters had been appointed to manage their own areas and liaise with one or two others. Assistant Directors of Nursing Services were appointed in support posts to assist the sisters and Directors of Nursing Services. Sisters were given the authority to manage their own areas and had direct access to the Director of Nursing Services.

Authority and supportive hierarchies

Batey and Lewis (1982) define authority as '. . . the rightful (legitimate) power to fulfil a charge (responsibility).' (p.14.)

It has already been noted how lecturer practitioners themselves have been invested with the authority to manage their own clinical areas with minimal interference. A further component of the restructuring of the organization has been to enhance the authority inherent in the roles of practising nurses. The development of this authority has taken place through the adoption of modes of care organization which emphasize nurses' taking responsibility for the decisions that they make and the care that they give. However, such authority would be difficult to employ without the knowledge to underpin such decisions. The issue is, therefore, one of allowing nurses the authority to make decisions and ensuring that they are equipped to make them:

'The more explanatory knowledge a nurse has and can use [author's emphasis] the more likely she is to have fewer problems in authority connected with practice responsibilities which she takes.' Batey and Lewis (1982, p.14.)

Devolving authority in this way can be seen as having a threefold effect. Firstly, it facilitates the development of professional practice. Professional practice is taken to mean a way of working where the practitioner works independently, using her/his professional judgement and exercising discretion in the way in which she/he does things (Vaughan and Pillmoor, 1989). Secondly, it has the effect of reducing the amount of direct supervision required from the leader of the nursing team. Finally, if the aim of an educational programme is to prepare professional nurses, it seems inconsistent to professionalize their training and to leave their learning environments unchanged. Otherwise, potentially, the problems of 'reality shock' (Kramer, 1974) will reoccur.

The means by which practising nurses' authority has been enhanced can be illustrated by reference to Ryan's (1989) notion of a support hierarchy. Traditionally, nursing was run along lines which Ryan (1989) describes as a command hierarchy. A command hierarchy is orientated towards achieving a quantifiable workload, co-ordination of work is by means of supervision by hierarchical superiors to whom workers are accountable. Work is routinized and difficult to change. It needs only a few trained staff to make it work. Ryan sees this model as being antithetical to emerging notions of professional nursing care.

A support hierarchy has as its objective quality care for its clients. The control of events is ideally vested in the client. The provider of the service (the practitioner) is accountable to the client. The practitioner is supported by senior colleagues who act as resources and facilitators, educators, associates, learners and ancillary staff. She/he works in collaboration with other members of the multi-disciplinary team. In effect, the pyramidal nature of a hierarchy, with leaders on top and workers as the base, is turned on its head. The resources of the organization are employed to support the practitioner in her/his encounters with clients. The above description constitutes an ideal type and does not correspond exactly to real life, for example the complexity of nursing work being client-led has been discussed at length (Brearley, 1990). However, as he himself acknowledges,

Ryan's work bears a strong resemblance to the ways in which nurses are working in Oxford Health Authority.

The lecturer practitioner and nursing practice

In the job description that she wrote for herself, FitzGerald (1989) sets a target of working on her ward uninterrupted by teaching or administration for one and a half shifts a week. This target can be met flexibly. The lecturer practitioner can fulfil the commitment on a weekly basis, or she/he can combine it to make three shifts a fortnight or six a month as allowed or dictated by other commitments. The practise commitment can be worked around other aspects of the role as necessary. On some days it may mean arriving on the ward before a meeting to care for a primary patient. Another day it may mean acting as an associate nurse for other primary nurses, or covering for a team to allow them time to have a meeting.

The clinical aspect of the lecturer practitioner's role includes acting as consultant to the ward team (FitzGerald, 1989) either through sharing knowledge or through helping nurses work through difficult situations. Practising alongside the ward team enhances the credibility of the lecturer practitioner. It also forms part of the supportive aspect of the role as well as providing clinical leadership for colleagues.

The lecturer practitioner and nurse education

As well as being manager of a clinical situation, the lecturer practitioner is a full member of the Department of Health Care Studies within Oxford Brook University. She/he therefore has responsibilities towards the development of the whole course. Lecturer practitioners are particularly involved in the preparation and support of clinical mentors and strategies for the assessment of student's clinical practice (Vaughan, 1990; Champion, 1992a). They head, plan and run the practice modules and, in conjunction with students and mentors, grade clinical competence.

The lecturer practitioners have responsibility for contributing to the planning of identified units within the degree programme, teaching on those units and assessing the performance of students. They also evaluate the teaching within their own clinical sphere. The planning of the educational experience of students in the unit takes place in conjunction with a course-planning team committed to facilitating the achievement of learning objectives relating to theory and practice as identified in the course curriculum (Vaughan, 1990).

The close supervision of all the students on a clinical placement in a lecturer practitioner's area would be impractical. In common with the national boards, the notion of the role of mentor has been adopted (English National Board, 1987). Since the term is acknowledged as being inexactly defined and employed (e.g. Burnard, 1990; Donovan, 1990; Morle, 1990) the notion of mentorship as employed in Oxford is discussed here. Mentorship has been defined as: '. . . an intense relationship calling for a high degree of involvement between a novice in a discipline and a person who is knowledgeable and wise in that area.' (May *et al*, 1982, cited in Donovan 1990, p.294.)

However, elements of choice on the part of the learner (they are allocated a mentor), emotional ties and continued sponsorship throughout the learning career as advocated in the works of, for example, Darling (1984) are at present diluted by the practicalities of the situation, for example, the brevity of clinical placements and the brief preparation of mentors.

The pattern of mentorship that is emerging presently bears more resemblance to the notion of preceptorship described by Chickerella and Lutz (1981) cited in Morle (1990): '. . . an individualized teaching/learning method in which each student is assigned to a particular preceptor . . . so that she can experience day to day practice with a role model and resource person immediately available within the practice setting.' (p.69)

During a student's allocation, mentors are supported and supervised by a lecturer practitioner. The experience of being a mentor is one from which the mentors themselves learn since they are required to be able rationalize their practice and to reflect on it. The present system can be seen to address the continuing challenge of moulding theory and practice together by involving clinically based staff in supportive relationships with learners.

The continuing education of practising nurses is given considerable emphasis. This, it can be argued, contributes to staff morale through allowing nurses to develop their own interests. It also contributes to the care given on the ward as the staff share their expertise with their colleagues. For example, on one ward, five staff nurses are on long-term part-time courses, one is reading for a higher degree, one for a Bachelor's degree and three for a diploma. There is usually at least one member of staff on one of the courses run by the hospital's post-basic education department.

Who are lecturer practitioners?

FitzGerald (1989) wrote that the exact qualifications of the potential lecturer practitioner were tentative. There is the issue of nurses who are well equipped to take on the role being unwilling to return to practice. As a result, the feasibility of allowing nurses with potential to develop into the role was entertained. Ideally the prospective lecturer/practitioner will be an experienced practitioner, manager, teacher and researcher, having a teaching qualification and a degree to denote knowledge either in nursing or one of the allied sciences. FitzGerald argues that once these jobs become established within the institution, nurses will not seek promotion by concentrating on administration or education and there will be more nurses who plan their careers to gain the necessary experience for the role of lecturer/practitioner.

The advent of the role of lecturer/practitioner has not met with universal approval. Davis (1989) outlines a number of criticisms based on observations of previous attempts at changing roles within nurse education. Davis states that the managerial and administrative responsibilities of holding a senior clinical and educational post is too large for one person. Certainly at first sight the description of this job does appear too large. However, given the logical possibilities of the structural and attitudinal changes involved, the load can be lightened considerably. This can be an arduous and difficult process. It requires time and tenacity, for example, see FitzGerald's action research into the early stages of her own job (FitzGerald, 1989). The same author, some years later, describes the satisfaction of having built a team of nurses who are continually building on their experience (FitzGerald, in press).

In order to avoid work overload, identified by other holders of various unified roles (including joint appointees) as being a major problem (Wakefield-Fisher, 1983; Wright 1983; Bellinger *et al*, 1985; Emden, 1986), the restructuring of the organization referred to above takes place on the wards as well as in the hospital hierarchy.

While the lecturer/practitioner retains overall responsibility and authority for clinical practice, she/he delegates work to appropriate people (Vaughan, 1990) by:

1. Developing modes of care delivery through which nurses accept responsibility for the care of a group of patients, for example, primary nursing.
2. Passing tasks such as the off duty or the overseeing of annual leave and study leave to others in the ward team, so spreading the load and also giving experience to those working toward promotion. Another effect seems to have been that such jobs have lost their former 'senior' status.
3. Negotiating the employment of support staff, secretaries, for example.

Such delegation frees time for the lecturer practitioner to undertake such vital work as clinical consultancy and supervision, giving support and facilitating the professional development of the team. The ability to delegate work to such an extent however does seem to be dependent on the freedom to develop an appropriate skill mix of staff. Also necessary is the facilitation of an atmosphere in which there can be an ongoing dialogue about how the roles of team members change.

It should also be noted that while a lecturer practitioner is expected to have mastery of practice, education, management and research, not all these facets of her/his role require equal attention at all times. The role can be seen as longitudinal, with one particular emphasis (clinical practice, say) being succeeded by another, rather than all facets requiring attention at the same time.

Within a ward team, a clinical career structure develops within which team members can move through the various clinical grades assimilating new skills in patient care, teaching (through being a mentor) and management. Two personal impressions of the clinical environment that can result from working with a lecturer practitioner are, firstly, that the roles of the whole team come to incorporate elements present in that of the lecturer/practitioner; practice, teaching and learning, management and research (as part of diploma/degree courses), and secondly, the environment of learning and developing that is available to the ward team encourages staff to stay on the ward for prolonged periods (2 to 3 years).

Another misgiving expressed by Davis (1989) is that lecturer practitioner roles may serve to alienate other nurse teachers from clinical areas. He states that all nurse educators should be 'facilitating what they teach'. He goes on to say that an even greater disparity may come to exist between what is taught by lecturers in college if a different grade of teacher is responsible for education in clinical settings. It seems that there is an assumption that lecturers teach only theory, lecturer practitioners only practice. However, lecturers and lecturer/practitioners teach side by side. The latter are also deeply and authoritatively involved in the clinical area to the extent that they can ensure a degree of congruence between what is taught and what is seen and experienced. The practice modules of the Oxford degree could indeed be called 'Praxis' modules (FitzGerald, 1991). Within them, theoretical ideas are introduced at a time when students are spending time in a clinical area. Nursing practice is seen as being central to professional education, reflection as a process is central both to learners' and expert nurses' analysis and to learning through practical situations (Champion, 1992a)

At Deakin University in Australia, the clinical contact of all members of the nursing faculty has been ensured by means of the establishment of both lecturer clinician and clinician lecturer roles (Deakin University, 1986). The former teach for 80% of the time, while for 20% of the time they work as staff nurses maintaining clinical expertise. The latter are head nurses with an 80% clinical commitment and a 20% teaching commitment, and are acknowledged as clinical experts.

Lecturer practitioners in Oxford are paid for partly by the Health Service and partly by Oxford Brookes University. As with joint appointees in the past there is a possible consequence of 'divided loyalties' (Davis, 1989). Champion (1992b) emphasizes that while the lecturer practitioners in Oxford do have a dual accountability, their role is unified in the area of practice with the educational element 'arising from and locked into the practice role'. Associated with this are possible problems of not being accepted by practitioners and/or teachers and of being subject to the dilemma of conflicting institutional goals.

The possibility of divided loyalties undoubtedly exists. However, the degree to which it exists varies between individuals, their backgrounds (e.g. predominantly education or practice), the culture of the institution in which they work and the model of lecturer practitioner to which they conform (FitzGerald, 1991). For example, a lecturer practitioner who works as a senior sister will, by dint of her post, be heavily involved clinically, while a lecturer practitioner who works alongside a ward sister may identify her/himself with the educational establishment.

The lecturer practitioners are indeed employed by two distinct organisations. At a time of economic scarcity they are required to show that they represent value for money, both in terms of the provision of cost-effective nursing care and nurse education. Nonetheless, it should be noted that senior nurses within Oxford Health Authority were instrumental in the establishment of the Oxford degree course.

The ownership of the curriculum development is seen as being equal between Oxford Brookes University Department of Health Care Studies and the nursing/midwifery services of Oxfordshire Health Authority (Champion, 1992a). As a result there are, to an extent, shared goals in what the two organisations are seeking to achieve. The lecturer practitioner's role can also be seen as one which seeks to bring together the conflicting demands of service and education.

In terms of their credibility in the eyes of clinical nurses, lecturer/practitioners can said to be aided by the fact that their teaching emanates from the clinical areas in which they themselves are directly and consistently involved.

CONCLUSION

At the end of the first part of this paper it was argued that the theory–practice gap referred to in nursing was one that exists between certain ways of seeing theory and practice; that is to say, theory, which is for various reasons irrelevant to practice, and a way of seeing practice which views it as inferior to theory rather than a source from which theory can grow and be refined. It has been further argued that the balance can be redressed through the development of practice and the revision of nurse education.

Throughout the mid- to late 1980s in Oxford Health Authority the structure within which nursing is practised has been changed, as has the preparation of new nurse practitioners. Central within this restructuring has been the evolution of the role of lecturer practitioner. The role seeks to unify previously separate areas of nursing endeavour – practice, education, management and research – within one role. The establishment of these roles involved the development of clinical areas for undergraduates from the Oxford Brookes University nursing degree. The main responsibilities of the lecturer practitioner are twofold:

1. To identify and maintain the standards of practice and policies within a defined clinical area
2. To prepare and contribute to the educational programme of students in relation to the theory and practice of nursing in that unit (Vaughan, 1990).

In terms of nursing practice this has meant the examination and development of notions of authority, support and knowledge in order to devolve decision making to practising nurses. In terms of nursing education it has meant locating the learning of the 'knowing how' theory in the same place as the 'knowing that' of practice (Vaughan, 1990).

REFERENCES

Alexander, M.F. (1983) *Learning to Nurse: Integrating Theory and Practice.* Churchill Livingstone, Edinburgh.

Allen, D.G. (1985) Nursing research and social control: alternative models of science that emphasise understanding and emancipation. *Image: The Journal of Nursing Scholarship*, 17(2), 58–64.

Balogh, R. and Bond, S. (1984) An analytical study of a joint clinical teaching/service appointment on a hospital ward. *International Journal of Nursing Studies*, 21(2), 81–91.

Batey, M.V. and Lewis, F.M. (1982) Clarifying autonomy and accountability in nursing service: part 1. *Journal of Nursing Administration*, 12(9), 13–18.

Beckstrand, J. (1978). The need for a practice theory as indicated by the knowledge used in the conduct of practice. *Research in Nursing and Health*, 1(4), 175–9.

Bellinger, D., Reid J. and Sanders, D.H. (1985) Faculty practice policy. *Journal of Nursing Education*, 24(5), 214–6.

Bendall, E. (1975) *So You Passed, Nurse*. Royal College of Nursing, London.

Benner, P. (1984) *From Novice to Expert*. Addison–Wesley, Menlo Park.

Benner, P. and Wrubel, J. (1989) *The Primacy of Caring*. Addison–Wesley, Menlo Park.

Brearley, S. (1990) *Patient Participation: The Literature*. Scutari, London.

Burnard, P. (1990) The student experience: adult learning and mentorship revisited. *Nurse Education Today*, 10(5) 349–54.

Carr, W. and Kemmis, S. (1986) *Becoming Critical: Knowing Through Action Research*. Deakin University Press, Geelong.

Champion, R. (1983) Integration of theory and practice: an analysis of the issues in relation to pre-registration undergraduate courses. Unpublished paper given at AIDCN conference.

Champion, R. (1988) Competent nurse? Reflective practitioner. Unpublished paper given at the 1st International Conference on Nursing Education, Cardiff.

Champion, R. (1991) Personal Communication.

Champion, R. (1992a) The philosophy of an honours degree programme in nursing and midwifery. In H. Bines and D. Watson (Eds). *Developing Professional Education*, pp.27–34. Society for Research into Higher Education. Open University Press, Buckingham.

Champion, R. (1992b) Professional collaboration: the lecturer practitioner role. In H. Bines and D. Watson (Eds). *Developing Professional Education*, pp.113–119. Society for Research into Higher Education. Open University Press, Buckingham.

Chapman, P. (1990) A critical perspective. In J. Salvage and B. Kershaw (Eds). *Models for Nursing* 2, pp.9–17. Scutari, London.

Chinn, P.L. and Jacobs, M.K. (1983). *Theory and Nursing: a Systematic Approach*. Mosby, St. Louis.

Clarke, M. (1978) Getting through the work. In R. Dingwall and J. McIntosh (Eds). *Readings in the Sociology of Nursing*, pp.67–886. Churchill Livingstone, Edinburgh.

Clarke, M. (1986) Action and reflection: practice and theory in nursing. *Journal of Advanced Nursing*, 11(1), 3–11.

Darling, L.A.W. (1984) What do nurses want in a mentor? *Journal of Nursing Administration*, 14(10), 42–4.

Davis, J. (1989) Who or what are LP's? *Senior Nurse*, 9(10), 22.

Deakin University (1986) Nursing Degree Curriculum. Unpublished. Committee on Nursing (1972) Report. HMSO, London. (Chairman: A. Briggs).

NHS Management Inquiry Team (1983) NHS Management Inquiry. The Team, London. (Team leader: E.R. Griffiths).

Donovan, J. (1990) The concept and role of mentor. *Nurse Education Today*, 10(4), 294–8.

Draper, P. (1990) The development of theory in British nursing: current position and future prospects. *Journal of Advanced Nursing*, 15(1), 12–5.

Emden C. (1986) Joint appointment: an Australian study illuminates world views. *Australian Journal of Advanced Nursing*, 3(4), 30–41.

English National Board (1987) *Institutional and Course Approval Process Information Required, Criteria and Guidelines.* ENB, London. (Circular 1987/28/MAT).

Farnish, S. (1983) *Ward Sister Preparation: a Survey in Three Districts.* Chelsea College, University of London, London.

Fawcett, J. (1980) A framework for analysis and evaluation of conceptual models of nursing. *Nurse Educator*, 5(6), 10–4.

FitzGerald, M. (1989) *Lecturer Practitioner: Action Researcher.* MN thesis, University of Wales College of Medicine.

FitzGerald, M. (1991) Personal Communication.

FitzGerald, M. (1991) *Chapter in preparation.*

Fretwell, J.E. (1982) *Ward Teaching and Learning.* Royal College of Nursing, London.

General Nursing Council. (1975) *Teachers of Nursing.* GNC, London.

Gordon, D.R. (1984) Research application: identifying the use and misuse of formal models in nursing practice. In Brenner, P. (Ed). *From Novice to Expert*, pp.225–43. Addison–Wesley, Menlo Park.

Gott, M. (1984) *Learning Nursing.* Royal College of Nursing, London.

Greenwood, J. (1984) Nursing research: a position paper. *Journal of Advanced Nursing*, 9(1), 77–82.

Gruending, D.L. (1985) Nursing theory: a vehicle for professionalization? *Journal of Advanced Nursing*, 10(6), 553–8.

Hagell, E.I. (1989) Nursing knowledge: women's knowledge. A sociological perspective. *Journal of Advanced Nursing*, 14(3), 226–33.

Hardy, L.K. (1982) Nursing models and research – a restricting view? *Journal of Advanced Nursing*, 7(5), 447–51.

Hockey, L. (1983) Bridge building. *Nursing Times*, 79(22), 64.

Hunt, J. (1981) Indicators for nursing practice: the use of research findings. *Journal of Advanced Nursing* 6(3), 189–94.

Hunt, J. (1984) Why don't we use these findings? *Nursing Mirror*, 158(8), 29.

Hunt, J. (1988) The next challenge. *Nursing Times*, 84(49), 36–8.

Hunt, M. (1987) The process of translating research findings into nursing practice. *Journal of Advanced Nursing*, 12(1), 101–10.

Jarvis, P. (1992) Reflective practice and nursing. *Nurse Education Today*, 12(3), 174–81.

Kramer, M. (1974) *Reality Shock*. Mosby, St. Louis.

Kuhn, T.S. (1970) *The Structure of Scientific Revolutions*, 2nd edn. University of Chicago Press, Chicago.

Lathlean, J. (1989) *Policy Making in Nurse Education*. Ashdale Press, Oxford.

Lathlean, J. (1990) *A review of research in nurse education with particular reference to theory-practice issues*. Unpublished draft paper.

Leininger M. (Ed) (1985) *Qualitative Research Methods in Nursing*. Grune & Stratton, Orlando.

Lister, P. (1987) The misunderstood model. *Nursing Times*, 83(41), 40–2.

MacGuire, J.M. (1990) Putting nursing research findings into practice: research utilization as an aspect of the management of change. *Journal of Advanced Nursing*, 15(5), 614–20.

Meleis, A.I. (1985) *Theoretical Nursing*: Development and Progress, Lippincott, Philadelphia.

Meleis, A. (1987). Revisions in knowledge development: a passion for substance. *Scholarly Enquiry for Nursing Practice*, 1(1), 5–19.

Melia, K. (1987) *Learning and Working*. Tavistock, London.

Miller, A. (1985) The relationship between nursing theory and nursing practice. *Journal of Advanced Nursing*, 10(5), 417–24.

Morle, K.M.F. (1990 Mentorship-is it a case of the emperor's new clothes or a rose by any other name? *Nurse Education Today*, 10(1), 66–9.

Munhall, P.L. and Oiler, C.J. (1986) *Nursing Research: a Qualitative Perspective*. Appleton–Century–Crofts, Norwalk.

Ogier, M.E. (1982) *An Ideal Sister?* Royal College of Nursing, London.

Orton, H.D. (1981) Ward learning climate and student nurse response. *Nursing Times* 77(23), occasional paper 77(17), 65–8.

Parse, R.R. (1981) *Man-Living-Health: a Theory of Nursing*. Wiley, New York.

Paterson, J.G. and Zderad, L.T. (1986) *Humanistic Nursing*. Wiley, New York.

Pearson, A. (1983) *The Clinical Nursing Unit*. Heinemann, London.

Pearson, A. (1989) Theory and practice: strengthening the nexus in higher education. Unpublished seminar paper given at the University of Wales College of Medicine, 29th November.

Price, B. (1987) First impressions: paradigms for patient assessment. *Journal of Advanced Nursing*, 12(6), 699–705.

Rogers, M. (1989) Nursing: a science of unitary human beings. In J.P. Riehl–Sisca (Ed), *Conceptual Models for Nursing Practice*, 3rd edn., pp.181–88. Appleton and Lange, Norwalk.

Roper, N., Logan, W. and Tierney, A. (Eds). (1983) *Using a Model for Nursing*. Churchill Livingstone, Edinburgh.

Roy, C. (1984) *Introduction to Nursing: an Adaptation Model*, 2nd edn. Prentice Hall, Englewood Cliffs.

Ryan, D. (1989) *Project 1999—The Support Hierarchy as the management Contribution to Project 2000*. Discussion paper, Department of Nursing Studies, University of Edinburgh.

Schon, D.A. (1987) *Educating the Reflective Practitioner*. Jossey–Bass, San Francisco.

Schrock, R.A. (1973) No rhyme or reason: a clinical area identification project. *International Journal of Nursing Studies*, 10(1), 69–80.

Smyth, W.J. (1986) *Reflection in Action*. Deakin University Press, Geelong.

Speedy, S. (1989) Theory-practice debate: setting the scene. *Australian Journal of Advanced Nursing*, 6(3), 12–20.

Tilden, V.P. and Tilden, S. (1985) The participant philosophy in nursing science. *Image: the Journal of Nursing Scholarship*, 17(3), 88–90.

Vaughan, B. (1989) Two roles-one job. *Nursing Times*, 85(11), 52.

Vaughan, B. (1990) Knowing that and knowing how: the role of the lecturer practitioner. In J. Salvage and B. Kershaw (Eds). *Models for Nursing* 2, 103–13. Scutari, London.

Vaughan, B. and Pillmoor, M. (1989) *Management Nursing Work*. Scutari, London.

Wakefield-Fisher, M. (1983) The issue: faculty practice. *Journal of Nursing Education*, 22(5), 207–10.

Webb, C. (1989 Action research: philosophy, methods and personal experiences. *Journal of Advanced Nursing*, 14(5), 403–10.

Wilson-Barnett, J., Corner, J. and De Carle, B. (1990) Integrating nursing research and practice – the role of the researcher as teacher. *Journal of Advanced Nursing* 15(5), 621–25.

Wright, S.G. (1983) Joint appointments 3: the best of both worlds. *Nursing Times*, 79(42), 25–9.

Wright, S.G. (1989) *Changing Nursing Practice*. Edward Arnold, London.

5.

THE SEARCH FOR IDENTITY

'When outmoded images begin to shatter, both old and new alternatives compete for ascendancy' (Kalisch and Kalisch, 1987).

If readers believe with Aroskar (1980) that 'the significance of image lies not in its validity, but in the firmness and energy with which it is held, and the influence it exerts on actual behaviours', then the inclusion of a chapter on identity within a book addressing changes in nursing will not be a matter for debate.

Perceived images powerfully influence both role performance and role expectations. These images are inextricably linked with identity formation. It is sometimes said that nursing, as a profession, is evolving through a period of 'adolescence' towards 'maturity'. The period, as in human adolescence, must involve the search for a sense of individual and corporate identity. Atkinson *et al* (1990) state that 'it involves feelings about worth and competence, deciding what is important or worth doing, and formulating standards of conduct for evaluating one's own behaviour as well as that of others'.

Calhoun and Acocella (1990) see the self concept as being the product of learning, containing the three dimensions of knowledge, expectations, and evaluations. They go on to make some interesting comments on stereotyping, which may well be seen by some to be relevant to nursing. They state that stereotyping involves loss of breadth and accuracy of perception: that the person stereotyped is then locked into a limited definition of personality and abilities, which may then be internalized. The nursing profession might well concur with their statement that 'the outdated image is a ripe source of conflict'.

Haralambos and Holborn (1990), considering image and identity from a sociological perspective, comment that 'self concept develops from interaction processes. It is in large part a reflection of the reactions of others to the individual. If defined as arrogant, servile or respectable, they tend to see themselves in that light, and act accordingly. The way individuals define situations has important consequences. It represents *their* reality in terms of which they structure their own actions.'

Murray (1979) defines self-image as 'harmony between what one is and what one does'.

If the foregoing comments of behavioural and social scientists are true, and if the Committee on Nursing (1972) was also right when it stated that 'inherited images influence current attitudes and policies', then it is essential to explore thoroughly this aspect within nursing, and attempt to assess its overall influence on nursing development and consequently on nursing care.

Nursing, it is sometimes said, suffers from a fractured image. This is not helped by the divisions of opinion that exist as to what nursing actually is, or what it purports to do. To this can be added the seemingly interminable debate as to whether nursing is, or is not, a profession, and whether it should or should not seek to aspire to such a status. It should not, therefore, in the light of these difficulties, be a matter of astonishment that many nurses experience a sense of role confusion, coupled with the need to search for a positive professional identity and self-concept.

PAST IMAGES

Modern nursing has its historical roots in the Victorian era: a period of dynamic change and progress in many fields, but also a period associated with narrow-mindedness, complacency, and oppressive social norms and attitudes. Women constituted, in many aspects of their social and economic life, an oppressed group within that society. The Victorian deification of motherhood kept many women out of the mainstream of social activity, and society exerted powerful control by means of its demands for 'respectability', and its sanctions on deviance from the accepted norms of female behaviour. Nightingale (1979) herself wrote of 'cold, conventional oppressive atmospheres where satisfaction of intellect, passion and moral activity cannot be satisfied'. It was an era of male dominance in all the major spheres of society, a dominance that would not be easily, or quickly, relinquished.

Historically, nursing has been identified with a less-than-professional image, as many nursing, as well as non-nursing, writers have attested. Prior to the Nightingale reforms institutitional nursing was largely carried out either by nuns, or by women from the so-called 'lower orders'. Examples of the second group have been immortalized by Charles Dickens in his novel *Martin Chuzzlewit*.

These images, as Bedford Fenwick was to remark a little later, 'clothed in bombazine and redolent of gin, were by no means creatures of his own imagination, but distinct types . . . of women actually in existence, and who had stamped the profession of Nursing with utter contempt and ridicule, instilling into the minds of the public an intrinsic antipathy to hospitals, infirmaries and workhouses, and which will take the combined forces of knowledge, sympathy and refinement years to eradicate' (Bedford Fenwick, 1888).

Williams (1980) comments that the early public image of the nurse was 'so hard and so cruel that the name 'nurse' was held in horror and contempt'. Toynbee (1983) states that nurses 'where they appear in the pre-Nightingale literature are usually dangerous and fearsome midwives, and layers-out; cradle to grave harpies nearer to witches and undertakers than ministering angels'.

While some of these and similar comments might be seen as something of an exaggeration, there can be little doubt that the mid-19th century image of the nurse was generally somewhat negative. Whittaker and Oleson (1964) suggest that Nightingale, following her work in the Crimea, succeeded in transforming for ever that particular image of the nurse. From then on the profession bore her image rather than that of Dickens' Sarah Gamp. This served to raise the status of nursing in a period when such seemingly heroic activities as those of Nightingale appealed to certain aspects of the dominant value system then prevailing.

The story of the establishment of the first nurse training school in Great Britain by Nightingale is well known, and does not need to be repeated here. Suffice it to say, as Carter (1939) points out, Nightingale sought to restore to nursing the prestige it had once had under the religious orders, and to reinstate the ideology of altruism.

The perfect nurse, in Nightingale's view, embraced a concept of triple motivation; natural, intellectual, and religious. The training school regime was strict, protective, and authoritarian, bearing the traces of Nightingale's own religious and military beliefs and experiences. Abel-Smith (1960) suggests that Nightingale perpetuated oppression by establishing a school in which 'the religious zeal of Kaiserworth, the military discipline of Scutari, and the cultural patterns of Miss Nightingale's Victorian home all influenced the nurses' training'. Conditions, by modern standards, were certainly harsh, and the student drop-out rate was high.

Palmer (1983) suggests that, as well as reforming the earlier image, the future image of nursing was also cast during the Crimean period. A relationship to medicine and hospital administration was established that placed nursing below both.

Class divisions, sharply defined in Victorian society, were also reflected in the structure and social mix of the Nightingale School. Nightingale's concept of the ordinary bedside nurse was that of a member of the servant class. Hours of work, living conditions, and the uniform devised all bear witness to that fact. The qualities required in the nurses were those of good household servants of the time; namely restraint, discipline, and obedience. The matron and the ward sister, coming usually from the middle and upper middle classes, were obeyed in all things, as were the medical staff.

Thus a new image and identity was being born which was more desirable certainly than that which had preceded it, but which also contained within itself the seeds of future conflict. The image of the nurse at the close of the 19th century, according to Palmer (1983), was that of a 'subordinate, servile, domestic, humble, self-sacrificing, and not too learned individual'.

This image matched in some respects the Victorian image of the 'ideal woman', and nursing came to be seen as a highly suitable occupation for virtuous and dedicated women. It also came to be seen as 'women's work', and the family analogy continued to be emphasised in nursing literature, with all its implications in terms of patriarchal relationships. As *Hospital* magazine remarked in 1905, 'Nursing is mothering'.

This image was to cling to nursing for over half a century. In 1939 Carter wrote: 'Nursing has been secularized, but it has in its bones nearly two thousand years of submission to religious order. The urge to obey, to kiss the rod, with its obverse the love of power, are not absent in the modern world, and nursing, especially institutional nursing, tends still to be a refuge, conscious or unconscious, for the naturally submissive.'

A London matron of the early period could write, without fear of contradiction, that a nurse must 'never ask why', and as seldom as possible 'how'; be content to bear unmerited blame . . . not be surprised to find herself vehemently repressed if she ventures on the faintest suggestion, and especially if she is at all forward or clever.' She suggests 'that courage of endurance and the spirit of self-sacrifice, along with cheerful obedience are highly to be desired'. She concludes that 'no life is more hard to live nobly than a life of loyal servitude' (Mollett, 1888).

It must also be remembered, however, that the emphasis on docility and discipline also served what was seen to be a positive purpose at the time. The submissive nurse presented no threat to the doctor, and was therefore less likely to arouse strong medical opposition, while the emphasis on strict discipline represented a very necessary attack on the previous image of the nurse. However, as Abel-Smith (1960) points out, there was also the problem in the early years that little could be done to change the often appalling working conditions, owing to the limitations imposed by the image nurses had adopted: 'Underfed, over-worked, and underpaid they struggled on rather than break a "professional" code of honour. Activism was unprofessional, worse still it would have undermined the cherished spirit of vocation: it smelt of hard bargaining and the pursuit of selfish material interests. It was also unfeminine.'

The wearing of uniform also played a part in contributing to a certain kind of image. It became one of the symbols of nursing and, having strong traditional roots, it has remained so. It has been, and is, indicative of status within the nursing hierarchy. Writers have viewed the uniform issue from many different perspectives. Savage (1987) sees an association with service and submission. There is the suggestion that the wearer becomes a blank slate on which an identity can be projected from outside. Female uniforms can play an important part in amplifying stereotypes in ways that the male uniform does not. Rogers (1991) pointed out that some of the more highly traditional uniforms can be 'fussy to the point of actually being dangerous'. Uniform remains, to the present day, a somewhat contentious issue, as the debate on the introduction of a national uniform during the last decade has borne witness. Uniform, devised originally for the practical purpose of protection, also became in itself a symbol of distinction, varying from one training school to another. Designs, originally bearing a strong resemblance to the uniform of Victorian household servants, did nothing and, until recently have done nothing to enhance an image already cast in the servitor mould.

Seeds of future discontent within the occupation were sown in the late 19th and early 20th century period, partly due to the transmission and tenacious adherence by generations of nursing leaders to what were to become, as time went on, increasingly outmoded forms of authority, power, and discipline. In a rapidly advancing society the image had to change, and the profession, though fearful of change, sought nonetheless for a new identity. That search is still in progress.

GENDER INFLUENCES

Many factors influence the creation of an image. Some of these have already been identified within the historical context. Not the least powerful is that of gender. Savage (1987) comments that 'sexuality and gender are evident within the very structure of nursing'. They influence how nurses are seen, and construct the present-day images and attitudes, including those as disparate as 'angel', 'battleaxe', 'handmaiden' and 'sex symbol'.

Nursing, as Gaze observed in 1991, has always had a problem with its image. It is a predominantly female profession, which is inextricably linked to the position of women within society. As has already been indicated, the profession was founded during a period of male dominance. The early image of the new type of nurse had to be in tune with Victorian ideology as it related to womanhood. However, the feminist movement was also gathering strength through this period, and its influence would be felt in due course.

Feminism can be defined as 'a world view that values women and that confronts systematic injustices based on gender' (Chinn and Wheeler, 1985). There are four major philosophical approaches to feminist theory; liberal, marxist, socialist and radical. The basic tenet of feminism, however, shared by all these approaches is that women constitute an oppressed group. This may be of particular relevance to students of nursing.

An oppressed group, according to Roberts (1983), can be seen as 'a group controlled by forces outside themselves that have greater prestige, power and status . . .' Friere, (cited by Roberts 1983) sees the major characteristics of oppressed behaviour as stemming from the ability of dominant groups to identify their norms and values as the 'right' ones, and also having the power to enforce them. He goes on to point out that 'the characteristics of the subordinate group become negatively valued'. These norms then become internalized in both groups.

Group traits in nursing bearing a relationship to oppressed group behaviour include lack of self-esteem, lack of pride in nursing accompanied by a failure to support, or participate in, professional organizations. Other features sometimes demonstrated include displaced aggression (horizontal violence) towards colleagues, both at micro and macro levels of activity, control by others, and lack of autonomy. Leaders in such groups have also been noted as having negative attributes, such as being highly controlling, coercive, and rigid in approach.

Nursing from its inception has always been closely linked to 'femaleness'. According to Hunter (1988) this had its origin in the home where nursing was seen as a natural part of 'women's work': 'Nurse equals Woman, but even on a profounder mythological level, Woman equals Nurse.' She suggests that female nurses as characters in literature are *always* symbolic of Woman writ large. They tend to be romanticized, sentimentalized, or satirized, but seldom presented straightforwardly. She comments on the great gap that exists between fictional images and social reality.

Melosh (1988) suggests that 20th century literature tends to portray nurses as either icy martinets, sexual predators, or as threats to male prerogative; while Muff (1988) emphasizes the importance of how nurses see themselves, which 'colours their perception of events, determines their actions, and makes them particularly vulnerable to the damaging effects of sexism and discrimination in a male-dominated health care system. The dual socialization of female nurses – as women and as nurses – to traditional 'feminine' identification contributes to the status and power inequities in nursing.'

She points to the antecedents of stress in nursing, including professional socialization to compliance, submissiveness and dependence; also to the problem of educational isolationism, helping to foster the characteristics stated earlier, as well as those of authoritarianism and perfectionism. The seeds of dissatisfaction, she suggests, are sown in schools of nursing. In examining the concept of selflessness in nursing, related to the above factors, she points to the dangers of over-valuing others and undervaluing the self. Nurses, she comments, are often coerced into giving more than they are able in the name of 'duty' or 'obligation'. The cost of this is high; guilt feelings if they refuse, and resentment if they submit.

Fielder (1988) suggests that nursing is *the* archetypal female profession. Nurses are seen as both sustainers, and subordinates. In terms of female nurses caring for male patients, nurses are 'often portrayed as erotic figures of a peculiar, ambiguous kind', being both theoretically taboo and sexually desirable. When older they may be seen as asexual mothers. Conversely, they may also be seen as bullying, blustering or condescending. The writer suggests that the archetypes underlying these images are older than the profession, and as old as patriarchal society itself.

All the dominant stereotypical images of the nurse share one common feature, the nurse as female. Men, however, have entered nursing in increasing numbers over the past half century, even though they constitute only 10% of the workforce. Increased recruitment of male nurses has been called for more recently by both the United Kingdom Central Council and the National Boards, in order to defuse the so-called 'demographic time bomb' that the falling birth rate represents.

Images of the male nurse tend to suffer the same distortions and the same reality gap as do those of their female counterparts. Men in nursing have tended to be a contentious issue, often seen as either Casanovas or homosexuals. The idea of men taking on the traditional female role of caring sometimes raised questions concerning their masculinity. As Cottingham (1987) relates in his article on male nurse recruitment, 'you need to convince men that it's fine to be macho and caring'. Dingwall (1979) suggests that many male entrants may see nursing as a possible avenue of upward social mobility. Despite this, recruitment remains low in comparison to female entrants and, as Naish (1990) points out, part of the difficulty may lie in the fact that nursing as a female-dominated profession may be seen as less worthwhile, and that males who join it are seen to be to some extent emasculated.

Despite these supposed problems, the 10% of men in the nursing profession currently hold approximately 50% of top posts in management, education, professional organizations and Statutory Bodies related to nursing. Their contribution to the profession seems set to increase significantly over the next decade, taking an ever disproportionately prominent role in nursing politics and other professional activities.

Many female nurses welcome the prospect of increasing numbers of men in nursing, hoping that it will lead to positive improvements, such as the promotion of professionalism and higher pay. These hopes, however, have been accompanied in some instances by a fear of a male takeover. It has been argued, as Gaze (1987) related, that 'the emergence of men in many of the most influential positions in the nursing profession has led to a growing emphasis on a 'masculine' ideology of science, rationalism, and high-technology specialisms to the detriment of practical bedside nursing.'

However, Savage (1987) suggests that the *assumption* that certain qualities are predominantly masculine or feminine should itself be challenged. The idea that rationality is specifically a masculine trait, and that women are, by reason of having a greater emotional component to their make-up, less rational, may be seen as a highly debatable point.

There is little doubt that gender issues will continue to occupy a prominent position in nursing debate for a considerable time to come as differing professional ideologies fight for predominance. The importance of such issues in the moulding of new images and the search for a professional identity in the modern world remains indisputable.

MEDIA INFLUENCES

The mass media is a powerful channel for stereotypical distorted images, and nursing has suffered considerably at its hands throughout the 20th century. Stereotypes can be harmful. As Elms and Moorehead (1977) point out: 'what stereotyping does is catch people up in their own mythology. They begin to believe the stereotype and not see reality. Their expectations and explanations no longer relate to what is really happening in the world, but to what they believe is happening based on the mythology portrayed in the stereotype.'

One of the most extensive studies of nurses and nursing as portrayed in the mass media of TV, films, books, journals and newspapers was that carried out by Beatrice and Philip Kalisch in the 1980s. In their book *The Changing Image of the Nurse*, they comment that 'the mass media substantially influences public perceptions of care, particularly nursing care'. Image is defined by them as 'the sum total of beliefs, ideas and impressions people have of nurses and nursing'. They go on to point out that 'once an ideology has taken hold it expresses itself not only in clinical practice, but also at the highest levels of health care service, organization and structure' (Kalisch 1987).

The study indicates that portrayals of nurses in the mass media over the past two decades, in contrast with earlier periods, tend generally to be derogatory in character. Attention is drawn to the dangers inherent in negative public images; reminding readers, for example, that public opinion plays an important part in ensuring the success of social, political, or professional groups in attaining their goals. Negative images may distort the public concept of nursing, and reinforce outmoded beliefs, expectations and myths.

In addition to the above, the suggestion is made that such images may affect the quality and quantity of potential recruits to the profession. In regard to Great Britain, an examination of English National Board figures for the mid 1980s indicated falling recruitment. Though many factors have doubtlessly contributed to this problem, it would be unwise perhaps to discount media influences here. The majority of career choices are made early in life, when the influence of dominant professional images may be considerable. Distorted images may bring about false expectations and wrong choices.

The study suggests that media images also affect policy makers in their allocation of scarce resources, as well as influencing potential consumers of health care, depriving them of important knowledge regarding the range of services that are provided by nurses.

Nurses themselves may also be adversely affected by such distortions of their professional roles, resulting in damaged self-image, and an undermining of self confidence, beliefs and values. The Kalischs maintain that 'the quality and quantity of mass communications pertaining to nursing strongly influence the cause of the nursing profession by shaping the nature of nursing's relationship with the public it serves'. They suggest that there is an agenda-setting function here assumed by the mass media, giving rise to an urgent need for a transformation of the image of the nurse to one that emphasizes equality, commitment to a career, and renunciation of nursing as a physician-dominated occupation demanding an impossible degree of obedience. They suggest that the dearth of viable role models in the media only serves to perpetuate traditional images.

There would appear to be an urgent need for nurses themselves to intervene in this situation by voicing their objections more powerfully to demeaning or damaging media portrayals of their work. In the British context it is encouraging to note that professional organizations, as well as individuals, are now becoming much more aware of media distortions, and these are now being more vigorously opposed than formerly. The complaint put forward by a group of Cornish nurses regarding the description of nurses given in the 1990 *Concise Oxford Dictionary of Current English* as 'persons trained to assist doctors in caring for the sick or infirm' is a case in point. Their clearly articulated protest will hopefully bring about a change of definition in the next edition of that work (Hobson 1992).

The Kalisch study referred to above deals particularly with the North American situation, where the bulk of their research studies were carried out. However, many of the problems they draw attention to have parallels within the British nursing context and are therefore worthy of consideration. As Clay (1987) commented: 'It matters not a jot that nurses are becoming better able to argue their case, to feel comfortable with using research, to extend and develop their role, if the media continue to distort and misrepresent their work.'

Not all writers and researchers into images of nurses within the mass media, however, would necessarily support all that the aforementioned writers have suggested. Hughes' study in 1980, examining images as portrayed in popular magazines, novels and newspapers 1976–86, showed that generally nursing *was* understood by the public at large. Andrews, quoted in the same study, suggests that 'the public forms its image on the basis of personal contact, rather than media portrayals'.

The present author tends to feel that probably both influences are at work, one shaping, moulding, or modifying the other. This conviction arises out of numerous experiences as a ward sister during the period when *Emergency Ward 10* was enjoying great popularity. One example from many will suffice for illustration. The author was engaged in running a very busy ward, where chronic staff shortage kept all 'on the run' continually. One surprised patient commented one day that he never realized that sisters actually worked, 'I thought they stood with their arms folded directing others, like they do on *Emergency Ward 10.*'

Karpf (1988), who has also studied and written on media images in nursing, draws attention to yet another facet of the problem: 'Something curious happens to the media when the subject of nursing crops up: the tone turns distinctly rhapsodic. The 'angels' labels has been the bane of many nurses for years, and reporters are inclined to treat nurses as if they were unqualified geysers of nurturance rather than staff working at full tilt under pressure.'

The 'angel' label appears to be a bone of contention, not only because of the potential it carries for sentimentalizing or trivializing what, in reality, is often a challenging and difficult role, but also because of the characteristics that frequently accompany the label. Salvage (1985) comments that the 'angel' is usually seen as 'compliant, willing, caring, dedicated, and invariably female'. Hughes (1980) sees the 'angel' as being perceived as a 'born nurse'. One is reminded here of the comment made by the Committee on Nursing (1972) that "born not made" is perhaps the most stubborn of all the stereotypes'.

The consequences of the 'angel' image for nurses is summed up by Minghella (1983): '. . . the notions of vocation, self-sacrifice and philanthropic benevolence implicit in these stereotypes perpetuate the view that pay is irrelevant compared with the privilege and satisfaction of doing good for others. Any suffering which nurses experience actually adds to their virtue.'

It has to be admitted also that very often nurses make little effort themselves to counteract the 'angel' image, being 'secretly flattered by the idea that they are selfless and dedicated, they do little to shatter the stereotype' (Bridges, 1990). Salvage, writing in 1983, suggested that 'the images not only deny her hardboiled pragmatism and political shrewdness, their repetition devalues dedication and altruism'.

In contradistinction to the above difficulty, nurses have also been portrayed as cruel, sadistic and malevolent. A well known example here is the character of Nurse Ratched in *One Flew Over the Cuckoo's Nest.* The battleaxe image, though now seemingly fading, has been a popular target for satirists in the media, as portrayed by the late Hattie Jacques in the *Carry On* films. These ladies are almost invariably spinsters, and it has been suggested that the abuse of power often demonstrated might act as some form of consolation for failure to attain to marriage and motherhood. Feminist writers of course might offer another explanation! The important point at issue, however, must surely be 'that breaking the vicious circle of media-created images is the central task facing nurses' (Naish, 1990). Probably few would disagree with Naish's statement. On a more hopeful note it should be borne in mind that recent media portrayals of nurses and nursing now appear to be approximating more closely to reality, and also providing more positive portrayals of men in nursing. *Casualty* and *Jimmy's* could perhaps be cited as examples of this trend.

THE HANDMAIDEN

Just as distorting as some media images is the image of the nurse as handmaiden. The handmaiden image, rooted in the Nightingale era, still survives in the 1990s. Nurses have always been trained to 'do as they were told'. Oakley, in 1984, bemoaned Florence Nightingale's emphasis on obedience in nurse training, commenting that 'had she trained her lady pupils in assertiveness rather than obedience, perhaps nurses would be in a different place now'.

Keddy comments that 'a look into nursing's history confirms that there has been an evolution of conflict between the nursing and medical professions' (Keddy *et al* 1986). Being a 'good nurse' invariably meant 'doing what the Doctor ordered'. Raisler (1974) suggested that a physician would judge a nurse to be good if she helped him, regardless of the patient care outcome. Any show of intelligence and judgement on the nurse's part is not seen as useful unless it improves the doctor's self-concept and feeling of authority. Stein (1967) wrote more fully around the topic in his study entitled *The Doctor–Nurse Game*.

Hunt (1984) notes that, unfortunately, nurses are still too biddable and submissive: 'What we have to learn is to become assertive (though not aggressive)'. This is further supported by McCarthy, writing in 1990, who comments that 'the status of nurses as underlings, independent workers subject to organizational and medical whims, creates morale and image problems at work, and dampens enthusiasm for professional nursing practice among practising nurses'. Champion *et al* (1987) add that '. . . if nursing is to improve its professional image it must address the issue of being perceived as powerless'.

Doctors themselves have traditionally regarded the nurse as occupying something akin to a servant role. Gamanikow (1978) points out that 'the division of labour between nursing and medicine, which mapped out nursing spheres of competence, was not a neutral division based on equal contributions to, and participation in, the healing process. Instead it created stratified health care and inter-professional inequality.'

Chapman observed in 1977 that 'although doctors want intelligent observers and a nurse capable of carrying out complicated technical skills in an efficient manner, most do NOT want a colleague in the true sense of the word. The emergence of the highly qualified nurse, in particular those with a degree, has been seen as a threat to their monopoly of knowledge and hence power.' She goes on to point out that many nurses themselves are 'loath to let go of their dependence on medical practice. Much of their status in the past has resulted from their association with the medical profession'.

The collegial relationship of mutual respect for another discipline, as McFarlane was to comment nearly a decade later, is an 'infrequent experience' (McFarlane, 1985). At the present time however, the shifting emphasis from curing to prevention and caring would seem to be indicative that as the 20th century draws to its close no ONE profession will have total responsibility for care.

As the demand for better educated nurses continues, in order to meet the needs of a society advancing rapidly in terms of medical science and technology, the transition from a relationship of submissive handmaiden to that of articulate, assertive colleagueship becomes an evermore essential ingredient of holistic patient care in the future. Unfortunately, as Canham (1982) points out, 'Nursing has a history of consent and humility which is perpetuated in its training methods'.

Marriner (1978) draws attention to the fact that leadership also poses problems in nursing. She comments that 'Schools of Nursing have placed little emphasis on teaching leadership, and what education has been offered has often been taught in an apprenticeship manner. The autocratic leadership style, so widely prevalent in nursing, does not foster leadership in others. Instead it contributes to an attitude that nurses are paid to follow orders rather than think.'

It would appear that the profession still has some way to go in setting this particular aspect of its house in order.

THE EVOLVING SITUATION

Austin (1977) comments that in no other occupation does a single title embrace such a wide spectrum of activities, from the very basic, which she describes as 'dirty and undramatic', to the highly prestigious. She maintains that central to an ideologically sustained consciousness is the image of the bedside nurse; a powerful image legitimating the single referent of 'nurse' shared by such a wide range of disparate groups. Wright (1991) states that 'Articulating what nursing encompasses, both to ourselves and others, is one of the most important tasks ahead of us'. He goes on to say that 'Unless we can say what nursing is, we are in a poor position to determine the nature of the role of those who help us'. McCarthy (1990) also warns that 'while parameters of nursing remain blurred then the threat of being replaced by technicians or the untrained persists'. She further adds that 'The level of autonomy as illustrated by substitution reflects the perspective that nursing is undervalued and unrecognised, and yet compliant and unprotesting'. Earlier work reviewed in this chapter would seem to support McCarthy's position.

Early history demonstrates that 'nursing' has been very much bound up with 'women's work' and being female. Nightingale took advantage of women's societal position and the Victorian view of 'women's work' when laying the foundations of nursing as a respectable occupation. Male recruitment at that time could have threatened nursing's subordinate role in relation to the medical profession in a way that female recruitment did not. Austin suggests that population changes, as they affected available labour through the period, also served to exacerbate sex and gender distinctions in nursing.

Garvin, writing in 1976, states that 'A changing profession in a changing society
needs individuals, males and females, who value the empirical, critical, and rational orientation'. Austin (1977) suggested that powerful sections of the nursing profession were encouraging the acceptability of masculine imagery as a rival orthodoxy. However, the problem arose that while feminine bedside imagery

matched nursing's professional ideology, masculine nursing ideology was out of step with the continuing predominance of feminine nursing imagery.

The advent of the Salmon Report and its implementation ushered in scientific male management. The latter had been the subject of criticism in the Report. Carpenter (1977) suggests that social-class domination of women in nursing was now being replaced by sex domination of men over women. The percentage of men in top posts mentioned earlier in the chapter would seem to support this contention.

Austin (1977) comments that it is very much open to doubt whether specialist, expert, impersonal and more bureaucratic nursing is in the interests of high standards of patient care. More recent developments in the National Health Service might lead one to consider that it is indeed right to entertain such doubts. She concludes a searching paper by considering that 'while masculine knowledge in the wider societal context is acknowledged for its authoritative status, in nursing its therapeutic value has yet to be demonstrated, and its presence in the hospital's social organization is widely seen as disruptive.'

The public image of the nurse today still tends to be that of a young, white, generally middle-class female. But this image is not true to life, any more than other images addressed in this chapter. There are now considerable numbers of older nurses, male and female, and nurses from a variety of ethnic backgrounds, all working in a range of varying contexts.

Darlene Hine (1988), writing of the North American situation states that black nurses face discrimination in employment from the very beginning: 'From the outset, the quest for image control and exclusiveness in nursing were essential components and characteristics of the professionalization process.' Blacks and lower-class whites were the most severely affected, being frequently denied admittance to training schools, and barred from professional association membership. 'By the mid-1950s', she states, 'the self-image of the black nurse was formed by the twin realities of racism and sexism'.

Recent research (Baxter, 1988; Carlisle, 1990; Torkington, 1987) suggests that the problems of racism and discrimination are also present within the British health care system. A recent report (Baxter, 1988) indicates that black nurses in Britain are aware of and unhappy about special difficulties at every stage of their career. Problems are particularly related to recruitment, deployment and promotion. The Report suggests that 'British-born black school leavers are reluctant to expose themselves to the humiliation and degradation endured by their parents and relatives, and that the number of nurses from ethnic minorities appears to be decreasing'. The question then arises as to whether nurses are able to provide good standards of health care to all sectors of the community if they are guilty of discrimination against colleagues from other backgrounds, thus contributing to the burden of a negative self-image for the affected individuals, and to the overall loss to the profession as a whole. One is reminded of Aroskar's comment at the beginning of this chapter.

IMAGE AND CARE DELIVERY

The public image of nursing, as mentioned earlier this chapter, affects the quality of health care delivered by nurses. Lindeman (1982) comments that 'the ability of nursing professionals to deliver health care is limited by nursing's image. It is thus extremely important for persons in the nursing profession to have an in-depth knowledge of their public image in order to maintain and/or improve their image and performance'.

Austin *et al* in their cross-cultural survey of nursing image (1985) noted that both 'nurse' and 'feminine' were perceived by their respondents to be 'good and active, but weak'. They suggest that the contemporary image of nursing has not changed greatly from the past. The image of nursing has not kept pace with the actual practice of nursing. The circumscribed, somewhat old-fashioned view of nurses and nursing that still persists reduces the ability of nurses to participate to the fullest extent possible in meeting the health care needs of society. As Hughes (1980) points out: 'Nursing potential has not been fully recognized or utilized by the public, and this has led to wasted nursing talent and inadequate care for society'.

Austin goes on to point out that 'the close link between 'nurse' and 'feminine' does raise some interesting questions as nursing sets out to change its image. Are nursing and female characteristics closely linked bbecause most nurses are female? Or is the practice of nursing so related to the act of mothering that nursing will always be linked to female characteristics? Can nursing change its image without a similar change in the feminine image?'

Will the female image be strengthened as more and more women enter traditional masculine professions? Will more men in nursing weaken the relationship between nursing and the feminine image?

These questions raised by Austin and others have significance for the future image of nursing as it enters the 21st century. As the writers state in concluding their study, the image of nursing must move from that of being weak and dependent to that of being strong and independent 'so that nurses can function effectively both in independent and inter dependent roles'.

Perhaps the comments of Hammer and Tufts (1985) need to be recalled by nurse educators at the present time: 'Nurse educators hold a vital key to changing the image of nursing in a very positive and permanent way'. They suggest that this can be achieved via more stringent student selection initially, and a display of genuine respect for the student as a prelude to the development of a healthy professional image and positive relationships with the service sector. They conclude by stating that 'rigidity, tenacious clinging to outdated practices, and the authoritarian role must go'. Although the writers were addressing the North American nursing context, it would seem reasonable to accept that parallels within the British context do exist.

Recent reported experiences from groups of Project 2000 students appear to bear this out. Although in many areas these students are welcomed and supported in their clinical placements, and the learning milieu created is highly positive, many students, regrettably, have experiences in sharp contrast to this.

Tattam (1991) reported that in some settings 'Project 2000 students are unable to use their initiative or take responsibility in clinical settings because other staff do not want to alter their routines'. Hooper, quoted in the same account, states that: 'It must be acknowledged that in a significant number of clinical areas, students are meeting routinized approaches, with little scope for student-initiated contributions, or for them to demonstrate personal responsibility'. Obsessive adherence to task allocation remains very much in evidence.

Accounts in nursing journals also indicate not only the lack of co-operation, but in some instances overt aggression. 'Staff treated us with scorn and contempt.' 'An experienced trained nurse once spat on the ground in front of me upon learning I was a Project 2000 student' (Hobson, 1992). The healthy professional image, still as yet at the developmental stage, can only suffer harm in such situations; damage is inflicted on and by all parties to the conflict, and the standard of patient care must inevitably fall as a result. Indicators seem to suggest that a positive professional image still remains elusive.

IMAGE AND IDENTITY TODAY

Clay (1987) draws attention to a major problem in terms of changing nursing's image, that of the fact that 'the public like nurses the way they are – or rather the way they imagine them to be; a heady mix of the angel and the whore'.

Both these images are ultimately detrimental to the ongoing development of nursing as a profession in the closing decade of the 20th century. As the reality gap becomes ever wider, expectations and perceptions become distorted or suffer disappointment. This is particularly problematic in the field of recruitment, where many younger applicants' expectations are garnered from the prevailing dominant professional image. Reality shock and difficulties in personal adjustment not infrequently lead to withdrawal from training, and account for a percentage of student wastage. Thus it becomes increasingly important, in terms of the waste in human and material resources involved, that this problem be urgently addressed.

The role of the nurse in terms of her real caring function has changed and is continuing to change, as is the treatment of the patient. Forty years ago the majority of patients were nursed in hospital, and frequently spent long periods in bed, thus supporting the dominant image of the nurse as a bedside nurse. Today the majority of patients are ambulant, and community rather than hospital-based care is in the ascendant. Modern medical science and technology ensure that the duration of a patient's hospital stay is very much shorter than in the past, and that many treatments can be carried out either as day patients, or at home. The reality of care no longer supports the image of the beside nurse and therefore is in need of change. A new dominant image, consonant with reality, has to be found, and with it a changing professional identity.

Many might agree with Curran (1985) that 'The foundation of nursing's image must be built on each individual nurse's professionalism. Creating a profession replete with nurses who are competent, productive, caring and effective in addressing the public's health needs is the first step in improving the public's view of us.' She goes on to comment that 'Nurses should establish themselves as experts and avoid being humble, tired, or apologetic'.

Central to the proposition of changing professional identity is to seek to actively change the image of nursing held by many members of the medical profession as well as the public. As indicated earlier it would appear that many doctors resist the concept of colleagueship with members of the nursing profession. Yet the demands of modern patient care render the earlier relationship of obedient, unquestioning handmaiden not only inappropriate and undesirable, but potentially futile and dangerous.

However, in order to address the problem positively, nurses must, as McFarlane (1985) suggests, challenge themselves and seek to offer to the health care system 'a discipline which is complementary rather than supplementary to medicine'. The continuing pursuit of a unique body of nursing knowledge and the expansion of nursing research might be seen as steps towards this goal. Other promising signs include, as Gaze (1991) points out, the emergence of primary nursing, nurse practitioners and nurse consultants indicating that growing numbers of nurses do feel assured about their self-image and are determined to speak out.

Some observers might, even so, agree with Newton, writing earlier in 1981, that the public might be reluctant to accept the new autonomous professional role of the nurse because it is dissonant with the persisting more traditional ideal, focusing on nurturance, service and subservience. The growing emphasis on autonomy might dehumanize the health care setting, it is suggested, by eliminating the emphasis on human needs that are best met by persons imbued with 'attributes culturally typed as feminine: tenderness, warmth, sympathy and a tendency to engage much more readily in the expression of feelings'.

Also there is the feeling in some quarters that there needs to be a return to a type of communication system which clearly depicts accountability and authority, accompanied by dress codes and titles. Curran (1985) poses the question as to whether such a move is possible where first names only are used. She points out that other professions, including medicine, retain such titles, and suggests that nurses should consider carefully the messages they might be conveying in dropping their own.

McCarthy (1990) comments that images in the workplace are often complex and contradictory, but that they can be used positively to portray nurses as 'versatile, specialized and possessing broad-based professional responsibility', spending, as they do, more time with patients than any other health care group.

Perhaps one of the key contexts in which old images can be transmuted and new identities be developed is that of nurse education, despite the fact that the nurse has always been viewed as a 'doer' rather than a 'thinker'.

Chapter 2 has dealt in depth with the new developments in nurse education at the present time, and the concomitant problems inevitably accompanying such changes, some of which were briefly referred to earlier. It will therefore suffice here perhaps to be reminded of the warnings given by Cohen (1981) concerning structural and cultural conditions within the profession. Cohen points to a number of problems revolving around inter-relationships; these include the perceived lack of freedom to think or act unhindered by the expectations of seniors, accompanied by intolerance to student resistance. The danger of practitioners and teachers merely producing replicas of the previous generation presents an inherent danger, and slows professional progress. She comments that 'in a rapidly changing society replicas of mentors become dinosaurs' and advocates a climate of trusting tolerance; perhaps not easy to develop in a profession prone to ritualistic authoritarianism.

This chapter has addressed a number of image-related issues, and has sought to trace, though not definitively, a developmental progression in the search for a true, relevant and acceptable professional identity. Nursing still bears the traces of its fractured image alluded to earlier. Media images still need constant vigilance by nurses themselves if they are not to send out the wrong messages. The handmaiden role is still not without its adherents within the profession among those who find it easier to 'obey' than 'advocate'. Images of racism still abound, and the anti-academic bias is still far from dead, as protagonists of educational reform and their students continue to discover to their cost.

The warning given to nurses by Virginia Henderson in 1980 is perhaps still appropriate, and worth remembering here: 'It is easy to convince ourselves that we are pulling our weight in the world if we perform adequately in our niche, which can also become our very comfortable rut.' It is not difficult to envisage how, in such a situation, nursing would continue to be, in the words of one writer 'the profession of unmet expectations' (Barnum, 1989). Perhaps many thinking nurses of today would agree with Barnum that 'The future isn't ours to read, to forecast like a passive audience ogling someone else's vision. The future isn't ours to presage; it's ours to make, to make of it what we will.'

The old and the new alternative images are still competing for ascendency within the profession, as the Kalischs foresaw that they would. It is up to the profession itself to make the ultimate choices.

REFERENCES

Abel-Smith, B. (1960) *A History of the Nursing Profession*. Heinemann, London.
Alderton, J. (1983) The best nurses have the essential qualifications before they go to school. Or do they? *Nursing Times* 79(10), 12.
Aroskar, M.A. (1980) The fractured image: the public stereotyping of nursing and the nurse. In S.F.Spicker and S. Gadow (Eds). *Nursing: Images and Ideals*. Springer, New York.
Atkinson, R.L., Atkinson, R.C., Smith, E.E. and Bern, D.J. (1990) *Introduction to Psychology*, 10th edition. Harcourt Brace Jovanovich, San Diego.
Austin, J.K., Champion, V.L. and Tzeng, O.C. (1985) Crosscultural comparison on nursing image. *International Journal of Nursing Studies*, 22(3), 231–9.
Austin, R. (1977) Sex and gender 1. *Nursing Times*, 73(34), Occasional Paper 113–16; Sex and gender 2. *Nursing Times*, 73(35), Occasional Paper 117–9.
Barnum, B. (1989) *Nursing's image and the future*. Nursing and Health Care, 10(1), 19–21.

Baxter, C. (1988) *The Black Nurse: an Endangered Species.* Training in Health and Race, Cambridge.

Bridges, J. (1990) Literature review on the images of the nurse and nursing in the media. *Journal of Advanced Nursing*, 15(7), 850–4.

Bedford Fenwick, E. (1888) The development of the art of nursing. *Nursing Record*, 1(29), 395–8.

Calhoun, J.F. and Acocella, J.R. (1990) *Psychology of Adjustment and Human Relationships*, 3rd edition. McGraw–Hill, New York.

Canham, J. (1982) Towards professionalism: time to speak our minds. *Nursing Mirror*, 155(13), 50–1.

Carlisle, D. (1990) Racism in nursing. *Nursing Times*, 86(14), 25–9.

Carpenter, M. (1977) The new managerialism and professionalism in nursing. In M. Stacey, M. Reid, C. Heath and R. Dingwall (Eds). *Health and the Division of Labour*, pp. 165–93. Croom Helm, London.

Carter, G. (1939) *A New Deal for Nurses.* Victor Gollancz, London.

Champion, V., Austin, J. and Tzeng, O.C. (1987) Cross-cultural comparison of images of nurses and physicians. *International Nursing Review*, 34(2), 43–8.

Chapman, C.M. (1977) Image of the nurse. *International Nursing Review*, 24(6), 166–7, 170.

Chinn, P.L. and Wheeler, C.E. (1985) Feminism and nursing, Can nursing afford to remain aloof from the women's movement? *Nursing Outlook*, 33 (2), 74–7.

Clay, T. (1987) *Nurses: Power and Politics.* Heinemann, London.

Cohen, H. (1981) *The Nurse's Quest for a Professional Identity.* Addison–Wesley, Menlo Park.

Committee on Nursing. (1972) Report. HMSO, London. (Chairman: A. Briggs.)

Cottingham, M. (1987) Putting men in the picture. *Nursing Times*, 83(20), 28–9.

Curran, C.R. (1985) Shaping an image of competence and caring. *Nursing and Health Care*, 6(7), 371–3.

Dingwall, R. (1979) The place of men in nursing. In Colledge, M.M. and D. Jones (Eds). *Reading in Nursing*, M.M. , pp.199–209. Churchill Livingstone.

Elms, R.R. and Moorehead, J.M. (1977) Will the 'real' nurse please stand up: the stereotype vs reality. *Nursing Forum*, 16(2), 112–27.

Fiedler, L. (1988) Images of the nurse in fiction and popular culture. In Jones, A.H. (Ed). *Images of Nurses: Perspectives from History, Art and Literature*, pp. 100–12. University of Pennsylvania Press, Philadelphia.

Firby, P. (1990) Nursing: a career of yesterday? *Journal of Advanced Nursing*, 15(6), 132–7.

Gamarnikow, E. (1978) *Women's Employment and the Sexual Division of Labour: the Case of Nursing, 1860–1923.* PhD thesis, London School of Economics and Political Science, University of London.

Garvin, B. (1976) Values of male nursing students. *Nursing Research*, 25(5), 352–7.

Gaze, H. (1987) Man appeal. *Nursing Times*, 83(20), 24–7.

Gaze, H. (1991) Changing images. *Nursing Times*, 87(20), 16–7.

Hammer, R.M. and Tufts, M.A. (1985) Nursing's self-image – nursing education's responsibility. *Journal of Nursing Education*, 24(7), 280–3.

Haralambos, M. and Holborn, M. (1990) *Sociology: Themes and Perspectives*. 3rd edition. Unwin Hyman, London.

Henderson, V. (1980) Nursing – yesterday and tomorrow. *Nursing Times*, 76(21), 905–7.

Hine, D.C. (1988) They shall mount up with wings as eagles: historical images of black nurses, 1890–1950. In Jones, A.H. (Ed). *Images of Nurses: Perspectives from History, Art and Literature*, pp. 177–96. University of Pennsylvania Press, Philadelphia.

Hobson, A. (1992) Give us a break. *Nursing Times*, 88(6), 42.

Hughes, L. (1980) The public image of the nurse. *Advances in Nursing Science*, 2(3), 55–72.

Hunt, J. (1984) Do we deserve our image? *Nursing Times*, 80(9), 53–5.

Hunter, K.M. (1988) Nurses: the satiric image and the translocated ideal. In A.H. Jones (Ed). *Images of Nurses: Perspectives from History, Art and Literature*, pp. 113–127. University of Pennsylvannia Press, Philadelphia.

Kalisch, P.A. and Kalisch, B. (1987) *The Changing Image of the Nurse*. Addison–Wesley, Menlo Park.

Karpf, A. (1988) Broken images. *Nursing Times*, 84(20), 16–7.

Keddy, B., Gillis, M.J., Jacobs, P., Burton, H. and Rogers, M. (1986) The doctor-nurse relationship: an historical perspective. *Journal of Advanced Nursing*, 11(6), 745–53.

Lindeman, C. (1982) Promoting the Image of Nursing. *Reflections*, 8.1.

McCarthy, G. (1990) The image of nursing. *World of Irish Nursing*, 19(3), 8–11.

McFarlane, J. (1985) Nursing-images and reality. *Nursing Mirror*, 160(1), 16–8.

Marriner, A. (1978) Theories of leadership. *Nursing Leadership*, 1(3), 13–7.

Melosh, B. (1988) A special relstionship: nurses and patients in twentieth-century short stories. In Jones, A.H. (Ed). *Images of Nurses: Perspectives from History, Art and Literature*, 128–49. University of Pennsylvania Press, Philadelphia.

Minghella, E. (1983) With angels in mind. *Nursing Times*, 79(34), 45–6.

Mollett, Miss (1888) Discipline. *Nursing Record*, 1(9), 99–101.

Muff, J. (1988) Of images and ideals: a look at socialization and sexism in nursing. In Jones, A.H. (Ed). *Images of Nurses: Perspectives from History, Art and Literature*, pp. 197–220. University of Pennsylvania Press, Philadelphia.

Murray, R. (1979) Self-concept is the key for nurse managers. *AORN Journal*, 30(3), 430–4.

Naish, J. (1990) Hard-pressed angels. *Nursing Standard*, 4(42), 17.

Newton, L.H. (1981) In defense of the traditional nurse. *Nursing Outlook*, 29(6), 348–54.

Nightingale, F. (1979) *Cassandra*. Feminist Press, New York.

Oakley, A. (1984) The importance of being a nurse. *Nursing Times*, 80(50), 24–7.

Palmer, I.S. (1983) Nightingale revisited. *Nursing Outlook*, 31(4), 229–33.

Raisler, J. (1974) A better nurse-doctor relationship. *Nursing*, 4(9), 21–3.

Roberts, S.J. (1983) Oppressed group behaviour: implications for nursing. *Advances in Nursing Science*, 5(4), 21–30.

Rogers, R. (1984) The image makers. *Senior Nurse*, 1(6), 10–11.

Rogers, R. (1991) *Politics and the Nurse*.

Salvage, J. (1983) Distorted images. *Nursing Times*, 79(1), 13–5.

Salvage, J. (1985) *The Politics of Nursing*. Heinemann, London.

Savage, J. (1987) *Nurses, Gender and Sexuality*. Heinemann, London.

Stein, L. (1967) The doctor–nurse game. *Archives of General Psychiatry*, 16, 699–703.

Tattam, A. (1991) Growing pains. *Nursing Times*, 87(51), 17.

Tattam, A. (1991b) Rigid ward staff set back P2000 students. *Nursing Times*, 87(49), 7.

Torkington, P. (1987) Sorry, wrong colour. *Nursing Times*, 83(24), 27–8.

Toynbee, P. (1983) The ladies no longer have lamps. *World Medicine*, 18(11), 32.

Whittaker, E. and Olesen, V. (1964) The faces of Florence Nightingale: functions of the heroine legend in an occupational sub-culture. *Human Organization*, 23(2), 123–130.

Williams, K. (1980) From Sarah Gamp to Florence Nightingale: a critical study of hospital nursing systems from 1840–1897. In Davies, C. (Ed). *Rewriting Nursing History*, pp. 41–75. Croom Helm, London.

6.

POLITICAL INFLUENCES IN NURSING — DOES THE TAIL WAG THE DOG?

Bruce (THE BOSS) Springsteen's record *Born in the USA* blared out from the disco in a hall in Ealing. The night was my 40th birthday and my friends had decorated the hall with balloons and banners. The banners had on them 'Born in the NHS'. The crowd was singing along to the tune of Springsteen's music but were singing different words as I walked into my surprise party. Everyone there knew of my love for the NHS. I was 40 years old, the same year that the NHS should have looked forward to 'life beginning at . . .'. In 1948, a very famous year in the opinions of many, the Aneurin Bevan dream came into being.

Organized health care in the United Kingdom was to be funded by taxes, free at the point of need, from the cradle to the grave. This freed people from misery and suffering, and protected their dignity. Ordinary working people could have access to health care without fear of a doctor's bill that they could not pay. 'A free health service is a triumphant example of the superiority of collective action and public initiative applied to a segment of society where commercial principles are seen at their worst' (Bevan 1952). Although it was a wonderful achievement, it could not however be described as 'user friendly' and it certainly did not give the 'user' any control over treatment. Nurses also were not 'user friendly' and were not encouraged to become 'involved' in patient care. They were encouraged to obey orders . . . Those practices hopefully have gone! Nurses today are the patients' advocate, planning care with the patient, and practising the skills and knowledge that the new education has given them (see Chapter 4), working as a professional within the multidisciplinary team. This change is happening in many areas of health care, and has the potential to be put into practice throughout all areas of health care if nurses want it to happen and if politicians keep out of the decision making in nursing practice. You cannot talk about health care unless you talk NURSING . . .

'Good Health' is not just a toast. It is what every parent wishes for their children and it is what every government should wish and plan for its people. Good health care does not just mean provision of hospitals, doctors and nurses. It means quality housing, a clean environment, a quality of life brought about by a strong economy, and a society comfortable with itself. When health breaks down for whatever reason, a caring government provides a health service that is multi-disciplinary, highly trained, and skilled to meet the demands of the consumer. When possible, it returns the client back to the community able to meet the demands of daily living. Politics and politicians have the power to facilitate that process or to create chaos owing to lack of strategic planning, short-term economic policy, or just pure interventionist politics.

This chapter is being written during the most aggressive and rapidly changing period that the NHS has experienced. Nursing has never been more influenced by politics. Questions are being asked and consultative documents produced, which suggests that the traditional method of funding the NHS by collective responsibility via tax payments by those in work needs to be challenged. The UK Health Service was the envy of the world. The USA, correctly, is looking at our system with the same envy. Now, over forty years on, there is a need for re-examination and changes will inevitably follow. Changes in health care provision are necessary to meet the changing needs of the users of health care and the rapidly changing advances in medicine and technology.

I have often asked myself why I became involved in health and the health service. Whenever I ask myself that question the answer is always the same. It is because I have always been brought up to respect people, to defend human rights and be an advocate for equality, which is needed so badly in access to a high standard of health care. When I was accepted for nurse training I was very proud and excited to have the opportunity to be part of a team of people whose aims were the same as mine. I had periods of disappointment during my three-year training and not all members of the multi-disciplinary team shared my enthusiasm for equal access for all people, or that nursing was about advocacy and empowerment of the patient. However, the general atmosphere was one of care and support, even though many practices were based on a tradition that existed for the benefit of the staff rather than the patients.

At the present time, massive changes are taking place within the economy. The country is experiencing the worst recession since the 1930s, as well as the privatization of all major services, including the funding of health care services.

British nurses have never been portrayed as 'political'. In fact the word has only crept into the curriculum in the last decade. It is still seen as something that nurses do not become seriously involved in. Why are we so different from our American or Australian counterparts? The election of President Clinton in the USA was strongly helped by the American Nurses' Association (ANA) supporting his campaign. We are led to believe that Hilary Clinton, who has the responsibility for bringing about a fairer system for Americans to receive health care on a need basis rather than the ability to pay, will be lobbied by the ANA Prime Minister Paul Keating's recent re-election for the Labour Party in Australia was in turn influenced by the Australian Nurses' Federation. The medical staff in Australia were not, however, overtly backing Keating's campaign. But when the nurses, *en mass*, expressed their concerns about a more 'insurance-led' system of delivery of health care, the people listened to the nurses not the doctors, and voted accordingly. In other words, nurses exercised their knowledge of the system and expressed their grave concerns about the future of health care. They became politically involved, seeing this as part of their role as citizens, professionals, and advocates for patients.

I know from first-hand experience that nurses shy away from becoming involved in political campaigns in the United Kingdom. The traditional health unions do campaign and are very 'up front' about which political party they support. The Royal College of Nursing has become more openly political in the last decade and I would personally give much credit for this to the previous General Secretary, Trevor Clay. I believe this political openess gives leadership an opportunity to look at governmental influences in health care and nursing. We must build on this work and help our professional organizations and trade unions. They cannot be proactive and politically vocal if the membership is complacent and apathetic. We live in a democracy and in every part of the country nurses are living and working. Nurses becoming politically involved in every parliamentary constituency could be quite a force for change! Much work has already been done with regard to the image of nursing in the UK, and readers will be familiar with this. If nurses in the UK do not realize the effect that politics today is having on their practice they are fools; I want passionately to believe that they are not fools.

The history of nursing frequently shows quiet passive nurses carrying out tasks and obeying orders, not encouraged to think or ask questions about the politics of the day. Some of us would like to believe that the recent changes in nurse education will correct that non-political approach. Sadly, I feel that very little as yet has changed. How we deliver nursing care to patients in a rapidly changing health service will, I fear, not be decided by the nursing profession, but by expensive government 'think tanks' whose main aim is to cut costs, contract services out to the cheapest bidder, and de-skill care into a number of tasks that can be carried out by a cheaper unqualified work force. It is already happening. Aggressive management styles are riding roughshod over thousands of nurses, both junior and senior, dictating how they, as well as patients and clients, will be managed. This has a direct impact on freedom to practice.

In this chapter I intend to look at some of the political influences that will have a major impact on the future for nurses and nursing. It will centre on the political significance of skill-mix reviews, the debate over quality of health care and that between patient-centred or task-centred nursing, the empowerment of patients, unemployment of nurses and raising the political profile of nursing.

RE-ORGANIZATION OF THE NHS

'The national health service is safe in our hands,' Mrs Thatcher boldly stated at the 1982 Conservative Party Conference. An endless collection of statistics have been produced by the Department of Health stating that more money has been spent and more patients have been treated than ever before! We have more nurses and doctors, and all is well . . . How is it then that hospital and ward closures are commonplace, record numbers of nurses are unemployed, and although more patients may be seen, more appear to be re-admitted after rapid discharge from hospital? Prescription and dental charges (when available on the NHS) have risen sharply and waiting lists continue to grow . . .

The Government's argument for the massive changes they have brought about in the NHS was the introduction of patient choice. The reforms, known collectively as *Working for Patients*, were introduced by the then Secretary of State for Health, the Rt Hon Kenneth Clarke MP, QC. The reforms were launched with massive publicity, which was quite unprecedented. The venue was the Limehouse Studios in London's Docklands. Mr Clarke's arrival by boat, sailing up from Westminster, reminded one of the arrival of visiting royalty! The audience,

300 handpicked senior representatives from North East and North West Thames Health regions, sat in quiet anticipation. They had been given boxes of video and visual aid presentation packages, which they were to return with to a loyal workforce and 'cascade' down the information. The presenter, Nick Ross, who also presented 'Crime Watch U.K.' on television (a pure coincidence I am sure!) hosted the link up. 'Welcome to this unique event. This is the most radical reform of the NHS in its history. Secretary of State wanted you to see it and respond to it as soon as possible.'

The Working for Patients video started with a regal-looking Margaret Thatcher and an old Pathé News film of General Practitioner (GP) surgeries, child health clinics and chemists shops in the early days of the NHS. It concluded with lots of stirring music and propaganda, which one would not expect an audience of very senior health service personnel to require. Mr. Clarke was introduced and it was explained that more detailed questions could be put to him later – at the regional road shows taking place during the rest of that week. The advice was taken by the audience and only very polite questions were put forward. Perhaps Nick Ross's timing of the famous Sam Goldwyn quote 'I want my staff to tell me the truth, even if it costs them their jobs', was possible just a bit too close to home for most! Champagne corks popped in NHS Trusts throughout the land on April 10th, 1992. The Conservative government had been re-elected and all the new bureaucracy of accountants and managers could sleep easy in the knowledge that their jobs were safe and the hidden agenda could, within a respectable space of time, be gradually released onto a tired and naïve nursing workforce.

When I was a girl I used to watch a programme called *What's My Line*. For fun and what I like to call 'research', I play this game on people who do not know what my occupation is. Key words are Market Forces, Income Generation, Performance Targets, League Tables, Skill-mix, Tender, Contracts, Corporate Loyalty, Customer Awareness, Cost efficiency, Marketing, Performance Related Pay and so on... Do they ever guess correctly how I earn my living? Readers will not be surprised that they do not! Now some readers may be forgiven for assuming that we have a dinosaur nurse writing this chapter. Not true. I love change. I find it exciting and challenging. Health care nursing and the NHS should be open to the changing needs of the population and change should be delivered in a responsive and caring environment. So how come I am uncomfortable with the language of the NHS reforms? Could it be that the hidden agenda is telling me that the 1990s will see the end of nursing practice delivered to patients and clients with the quality, advocacy and holism that we are renowned for? Or am I fooling myself that that is what nursing is all about? Maybe we need to look at how we currently practice, discuss how we ought to practise and then go on to consider how politicians think, and have planned for how we are to practise in the future.

As was stated earlier, all organisations need to be reviewed, and the NHS is no exception. The title of the White Paper *Working for Patients* could not be argued with. The content is a different matter. It was sold to a trusting public on the grounds that more 'choice' would be offered to consumers or customers. The reality is very different; patient choice is being reduced. People are directed to those hospitals where managers have set up contracts, thus restricting their freedom to go where they want. Accountability to the local community for health care provision has been severely curtailed because two thirds of the directors appointed to run hospital and community trusts are businessmen, accountants or property developers possibly from outside the area. Most of these new managers are not health care professionals.

Competing for contracts and cutting costs has become a priority for them. It is assumed that a change in skill mix decreases costs, so obviously the new trusts are concentrating on skill-mix reviews. Professor Dyson (1991) was commissioned by the Department of Health to produce a paper; he has been widely represented recently in all of the nursing press, and is making some quite controversial statements, such as 'I have been sent by the Government and I am here to help you!' . . . which means about as much to this writer as 'of course, I will still love and respect you in the morning darling!' or 'the cheque is in the post!' Therefore, let us now address the thorny subject of skill mix.

SKILL MIX REVIEWS

What is skill mix? One definition, as employed by the DoH, describes it as '. . . the balance between trained and untrained, qualified and unqualified, supervisory and operative staff within a service area, as well as between different staff groups.' Optimum skill mix is achieved when the desired standard of service is provided at the minimum cost, which is consistent with the supervisory personnel and the maximization of contributions from all staff members. It will ensure the best possible use of scarce professional skills to maximize the service to clients (Nessling, 1990, cited by Bevan and Stock, 1991). The main assumption behind skill mix is that skilled (and therefore more expensive) nurses should not spend their time doing tasks and activities that could easily be carried out by less skilled (and cheaper) staff. As Buchan and Ball (1991) note, 'many students have concentrated on identifying 'non-nursing' duties currently performed by nurses and theoretically allocating these duties to cheaper ward clerks, porters and assistants, etc.' There appears to be some confusion over the distinction between skill mix and grade mix. Skill mix reviews are very much in vogue. Compared with a few years ago there has been a large increase in the research and literature about skill mix. The *DHS – Mix and Match* was a major publication in 1986 (Department of Health and Social Security, 1986) but very little was done about this document until a number of new interests appeared on the horizon.

The development of the new health care assistant (HCA) role, and the opportunity to gain a form of training has implications for staffing levels on wards and in the community. Many auxillary nurses and care assistants have never had the opportunity to develop their skills to full potential. We should be able to welcome training and developments in National Vocational Qualifications (NVQ) for many years. Staff below the 'professional' level have been exploited in the past, undertaking work far more complex and responsible than their training has prepared them for and for which they are not paid. Clinical grading has so far failed to end the exploitation of nursing assistants and auxillaries.

Changing the skill mix in the work force is one of the key issues in today's market-led health service. Throughout the NHS skill mix changes, often called 'reprofiling the workforce', are being implemented. The health care internal market places a much greater emphasis on the cost of services. As hospitals and other health care units compete against each other to win contracts, the costs of these services must be as low as possible if trusts are to win them. The main problem with most skill mix reviews is that they are primarily, and often solely, cost-cutting exercises. They adopt a lowest common denominator approach that attempts to compile the cheapest workforce that is consistent with minimum standards.

In theory skill mix reviews could result in a more qualified workforce being introduced; this to my knowledge has never actually happened. So far skill mix reviews almost always result in cheaper, less qualified staff replacing more expensive, better qualified staff (Bevan and Stock, 1991). Executive, Personnel Development Unit, Oct. 1991 warns that the 'ratcheting up' of staff will need monitoring and containing. This is a very explicit warning against having more qualified staff and giving greater training.

Quality is portrayed as being a big issue in the health service today. However, I would suggest that only lip service is paid to providing a better quality of service, as the Executive report points out: 'in fact quality is rarely given prominence in skill mix reviews. Value for money and cost cutting dominate the expressed estimate for most studies' (as cited in Bevan and Stock 1991). I would support the most efficient use of resources and securing value for money, but this should never be allowed to be at the expense of lowering standards and the fragmentation of health care. If we are serious about the quality of care provided it must not deteriorate as a result of skill mix reviews. We are aware that the standard of care aimed at is the minimum acceptable to the purchaser not the best standard possible. The burden of proof must be placed on management to show that standards of service will be maintained. It matters little to many managers what means are employed towards that end as long as they represent the cheapest option available. It has to be stated that many managers, most of them nurse managers, are under intolerable pressure and stress to 'stay in budget'. The way in which budgets are organised will influence any cost-cutting effects of skill mix, particularly when dealing with certain non-nursing duties. Skill mix exercises should be evaluating the service critically to see how improvements in quality and service provision can be made. It should not just be cutting salary bills at the expense of quality of care. Dyson (1991) forsees a cost-cutting situation where nurses can be employed on a more flexible basis to service the peaks of demand, without over-staffing the troughs of the day, thus 'where self-employed contractees prefer daytime work, it is possible to staff nearer to the trough and to cover the two or three half day peaks with self-employed contract staff'.

In their review of the literature on skill mix, Gibbs et al (1990) commented on the lack of research on 'whether patient outcomes are affected by skill mix of a nursing team, or whether the same patient outcomes can be achieved by varying skill mix combinations.' The current emphasis on cutting costs has meant that the effect of changing the ratio of registered staff to non-registered staff on patient care has largely been ignored. In a report for the Royal College of Nursing, Buchan and Ball (1991) comment 'whilst many studies (often of grade mix) consider the cost implications of substituting one group of healthcare workers for another, comparatively few include an assessment of the outcome implications of such substitution. At best, many studies assume no decline in the standard of care provided'. So how does skill mix work in practice?

The Government's Value For Money Unit (VFM) has produced a report on skill mix in two community unit trusts which was 'made available widely in the NHS to allow others to benefit from the experience' (Kelly and O'Leary, 1992). The value for money unit has been criticized for reducing the comprehensive care that district nurses carry out to a series of tasks that can be delegated to cheaper nurses. Issues such as quality and health outcomes merit little consideration in the Value For Money Unit report.

In the following skill mix reviews the number of G and H grade nurses were cut and replaced with B, D, and E grades. In First Community Health Trust (Staffordshire), 69% of staff were on F, G, and H grades – now 31% are. In North Mersey Community Trust G, and H grades accounted for 51% of staff. The skill mix review proposed that only 18% of staff should be on these grades. Staff on G and H grades were reduced by natural wastage, or put in lower grade posts with protected pay and/or redundancy. The training of new district nurses has been stopped by both trusts. However, the skill mix reviews in both these trusts depended on much criticised activity analysis methods, which the Northwest region/York study (see below) stated over-simplified the process of nursing and neglected quality of care issues. (Activity analysis methods examine those activities that need to be performed in order to achieve an objective in the best way possible. It looks at work flows, job descriptions and the skills required to do specific tasks).

The skill mix reviews in the above community Trusts have huge implications for other community units, where on average 50% of staff are on G and H grades. At the time of writing the new Care in the Community Act has not been introduced. As nurses, many of us are concerned about how future care will be delivered in the community. We are all very aware that changes will need to be made; however, I cannot believe that the experience and knowledge that district nurses offer to patients and clients within the community can be de-skilled in this way, especially at a time when changes in the acute care area will bring to the district nurses' practice more acutely ill patients. I would recommend that all community and district nurses read *Skill Mix and GP Fundholding Contracting Issues* (CDNA UK 1993).

DEBATE OVER QUALITY OF CARE

Skill mix reviews have over-simplified the complex process of health care provision and neglected quality of care. It is not easy to measure quality of care. It can and should be measured with great sensitivity that can detect graduations of change and it should involve consultation with patients. The NHS Management

Executive's own study recognizes there are 'limits to role changes, which are necessary to prevent dangerous practice' . . . Bevan and Stock (1991). It does also give some recognition to the 'adverse effects' on staff who undertake work outside their job description. Can we be satisfied with a recognition that it will accept reductions in quality as long as they are not dangerous? We must have more rigorous criteria. A recently produced Centre of Health Economic's study and the North West Region/York study provides such criteria. Both of these studies were conducted by *The Independent* newspaper and a well-respected health research consortium based at York University (Bagust and Oakley, 1992). The Centre for Health Economics (CHE) at York University was commissioned by the Department of Health to examine the relationship between skill mix and the quality of nursing care (Carr-Hill *et al*, 1992). The CHE report is a detailed and thorough examination of the relationship between skill mix and the quality of care. Costing £250,000, it was completed in August 1991 but for some strange reason its publication was delayed by the Department of Health until October 1992 – just by coincidence, after the April 92 election . . . dirty tricks? . . . surely not! The study found that HIGHER NURSING GRADES GAVE BETTER QUALITY OF CARE. The study states that its analysis only 'provides a minimum estimate of the importance of trained staff to the delivery of good quality care'. Four of the fifteen wards with below average staff costs also had below average quality of care. The depth and scale of the study means that it is currently the definitive statement on skill mix issues. The contraints of the length of this chapter does not allow me to go into detail on the findings of this report. The response from trade unions to skill mix reviews has generally been wary, because their concentration on cost cutting, their lack of regard for the quality of care, and their adverse effect on staff.

The following is an extract from a paper by the Union In Manufacturing Science Finance (MSF), 'We recognise that all jobs change over time, nor are we interested in the defence of traditional arrangements just for the sake of them. On the contrary, our principal concern is that the service provided by the NHS should meet people's needs and be of the highest possible standard. Changes in support staff can help professionals do their job more effectively . . . The priority, therefore, is to ensure that variations in skill mix do not undermine these principles. Any changes should be properly managed, should emphasise the importance of training, and should not be used simply as a way of cutting costs or filling gaps in current staffing levels. Skill mix should be dictated by the needs of the users of the service, and not by the pressure of the market.' (*Skill Mix in the NHS – The case for a Code of Practice.* MSF, 1992.)

To ensure skill mix reviews are guided by the needs of the users of the service MSF have drawn up a code of practice for trusts or health authority managers who are considering changes in skill mix. The document argues that changes should be for the benefit of the users. The Royal College of Nursing have also produced a guide for its members on skill mix and reprofiling. It is an excellent document and notes: 'Experience throughout the UK would suggest that exercises are often carried out in quieter, less politically sensitive wards and nursing areas. Staff involvement may be limited, and skill mix exercises are presented to staff at face value; the implications in respect of future roles and delivery of patient care are not often fully explained. Therefore, it is critical that staff and stewards play a full part in any skill mix exercise and set the agenda from the outset.' (Royal College of Nursing, 1992.)

We must never forget that quality in health care is paramount. All nurses, professional organizations and the health trade unions should recognise that the CHE study is a useful means of ensuring that more lip service is paid to quality and ensure that the practice about quality matches the rhetoric.

HEALTH CARE: PATIENT-CENTRED OR TASK-CENTRED?

Task-centred nursing operates within a hierarchy of skills, within a team that can consist of skilled, semi-skilled, and unskilled personnel. This approach enables staff to undertake a variety of tasks under senior staff direction. Qualified nurses have a supervisory role directing untrained and trainee staff who provide the more basic care. It has been argued that this system leads to a better use of resources, avoiding 'the potential waste of expensive training and higher pay when professional staff carry out lower level duties' (Bevan and Stock, 1991). I object to the word 'lower' level tasks. I object on behalf of all patients, and I object, as a nurse, that people who are not directly involved with caring for patients, who have not have required care from nursing staff themselves should make such outrageous statements. It is my wish that all of us stay healthy, and do not require assistance to carry on with daily living, but that is not reality. Let's picture the scene: a senior member of the Government, Region, Hospital or Community Trust becomes ill and requires care and attention within hospital or community. I know, and so do you, that the nurse who will give that care is likely to be experienced and qualified. Now a variety of reasons could be offered for that decision, but nothing can convince me, nor should it convince my profession, that what is perceived as 'good enough' for the majority should also be 'good enough' for the minority. Of course put another way, what we know to be 'good' for the minority is also 'good' for the majority.

No-one would chose to have their car serviced or repaired by an unqualified mechanic, or to be defended in law by an unqualified lawyer, or to have their medical needs met by the doctor's assistant. I certainly would never have my hair cut by an unqualified hairdresser. We may decide to have somebody unqualified do some minor repair to the house or the car, and more than likely, it would be very minor. They usually make it very clear that they are not qualified and there will be no 'comeback on me mate' if it goes wrong. We are usually prepared to risk this mainly because we want to save money, and sometimes it works out alright. But sometimes it all goes very wrong, and there is always someone around to tell you what you really already knew . . . 'you should have asked the experts', and we end up paying out more in the end to 'make it better'. Why then do some experts feel that it is suitable to care for people with less qualified staff and risk a lower quality of care? With patient-centred nursing, also referred to as primary or holistic nursing, qualified nurses plan and carry out care based on individual needs, with the patient as a partner and assisted by other staff. A named nurse has charge of specific patients. From this approach the key question is not how many qualified nurse auxillaries or health care assistants are needed, but rather how many patients can a qualified nurse give care to.

If qualified nurses are not encouraged or even allowed to deliver direct patient care, how are they supposed to gain experience? The value of that care can be seen as has been stated above. It has been argued that focusing on tasks results in neglecting the role of nurses in preventative care, assessment and decision-making. If nurses take on a supervisory role this leaves them with little time to nurse, which would prevent them from developing their skills. It is argued that unless nurses remain as direct care givers as opposed to supervisors, they will never gain the experience needed to lead and manage others (Seymour, 1992). We must challenge at every level task-centred care if we are ever to implement United Kingdom Central Council (UKCC) guidelines (PREPP), which rightly argues for the nurse to gain a period of support following registration. The nurse then enters a period of primary practice, proceeding to become an advanced practitioner, continuing to develop knowledge and skills until she/he reaches consultancy level.

When nurses do practise at an advanced consultancy level, it is 'political' and it brings about confrontation. One of the saddest aspects of nursing for me in the 1980s was reading of the closure of Beeson Ward, Oxfordshire. Unless we were part of that enlightened nursing experience we cannot really feel the despair that those leaders in nursing must have felt. Beeson challenged all traditional thought, and all studies showed that the nurses were successful with patient outcomes, and also successful with costing, as it seems these were comparable with other wards.

Politics came on the scene when the nurses were seen as being too powerful. They were making decisions on admissions and discharges. Patients were very much involved in the process of care which the medical establishment did not like. If money rules everything in the NHS why were doctors not told to accept? Or is it also to do with power – it usually goes hand-in-hand with politics. The nursing community also practises clinical leadership and many nurse practitioners past, present, and most definitely in the future, will face conflict and pressure when they practise at an advanced level.

It was revealed at the recent Practice Nurse Conference in Swansea that many practice nurses are working in totally unacceptable circumstances with minimal time allowed for study, with no employment contracts or job descriptions. It is not commonplace for practice nurses to have time off for professional study. The extended role of the nurse practitioner requires the nurse to have access to such study. Patients should be much more satisfied as a result.

In the early 1980s a general practice in Birmingham employed two nurse practitioners; the results can be read in full in a document titled 'Nurses do it better' workshop at AGM of ACHCEW 1986. Over the three years that the scheme was in operation an excellent relationship was built up between patients and nurses. All of those who saw the nurses said they would be happy to return and that they trusted them to refer them to a physician if necessary. They said that talking to the nurse was less embarrassing, better for advice, and that she 'will give you more time'. The nurse was prepared to spend more time explaining why a procedure was necessary and also 'listened' when the doctor did not have time. Eighty-eight percent of patients thought nurse practitioners were a good idea and appeared to be more user-friendly. What we need is a *Which?* magazine consumer guide to health care, and I confidently predict that it will say 'Nurses do it best'.

The Government's 'Patient's Charter' seems to endorse the patient-centred view of nursing, and therefore rejects the basis of most skill mix reviews. It states that, 'all patients should have a named, qualified nurse/midwife or health visitor who will be responsible for their nursing or midwifery care' (Department of Health, 1991). The former Director of Personnel for the NHS, Eric Caines, seems to believe that anyone can hold the hand of a dying patient. Does he not recognize the skill that is required to handle such sensitive care? He often states that patients prefer their 'ordinary needs' to be met by support workers. I have yet to be made aware of any evidence to back up these statements. Mr Caines has recently stated that at least 200,000 NHS staff could be sacked, and that this could come from nursing and medicine. He challenges the Government, and states that they are afraid to take on the nurses and doctors!

Mr Caines no longer works for the NHS – he is now a Professor of Health Service Management at Nottingham University. His students will presumably be future managers. I sincerely hope that they are able to challenge him with research evidence that make his statements worthy of nothing more than being controversial discussion points that are useful to stimulate debate.

Nurses should, and could, arrange public debates on the 'Patients' Charter' within their hospital or community. If it is working well it will be very positive for staff, unit managers and, of course, patients. If, however, there are shortfalls, we need to address the weak areas and work with all parties to improve care; be honest with the public, and inform the politicians that the 'Patients' Charter' is not being implemented.

When are we going to challenge what is happening to nursing and to quality of patient care? For example, amongst other things, we have silently allowed patients and staff to be charged for parking their cars when visiting the hospital. We have witnessed the 'patrol' workers ready to pounce on a distressed groups of people when their ticket has overrun. Even televisions are for hire in a large number of hospitals. How do we cope as nurses when patients and their families cannot afford to pay for these amenities.

Back-door privitization has been going on for some time and we have remained silent. The private sector is now coming through the front door, and has no respect for the professions. Recent events in the West Midlands has exposed exploitation beyond belief of taxpayers' money being used, for example, to hire private jets to fly American management consultants around the Country to give advice to managers within the NHS about cost-effective styles of delivery of care!

EMPOWERMENT OF PATIENTS

How can we, as nurses, enable patients to be empowered to speak for themselves? We need people to be truly involved in their own health care. If we choose to practise as caring professionals, surely part of that practice is to see that patients and potential patients are informed of the reality of the market led NHS, and that they understand what 'skill mix' in their hospital and community means. 'Nurses should unite to resist the silent bureaucratic dismantling of the National Health Service, which is the envy of the USA'. So said Professor Patricia Benner, Professor of Nursing at the University of California, at a nursing conference in Glasgow in September 1991. In an interview given to *Nursing Times* (Friend, 1991), she went on to say she was 'astonished by the changes that had taken place in Britain's health service. There is too much misplaced faith in accountants. The importation of the market and cost benefit analysis in a system that was exemplary is not very encouraging. I am hoping that nurses will have a vision of what is worth preserving. Across the Atlantic', she said, 'nurses were intent on trying to get a national health care system introduced'. She strongly warned against using the economic and strategic language of the new market system, as if this would bestow on them status and power that they do not have now. It was not an advance to 'trade in' the language of practice. 'I think they could unite and be very powerful and become more political about the silent bureaucratic dismantling of the health service'. Dr. Benner is respected within the world of nursing and is right to encourage us not to accept these changes without opening up the debate.

In the recent report referred to earlier in the chapter on private funding and contracts operating in the N.H.S. a kidney dialysis unit in Rotherham was run by a private company which had recently won the contract. Nurses have been trained in 'elementary' technical skills to reduce the need for separate technicians, and of course to reduce the cost. My concern centres on the quality of care, and whether the nurses would have less time for 'human skills'. Recently, when out with friends who had just returned from the United States, we discussed changes in health care. The discussion developed around quantity, and would it enable more people to be treated? I do not believe that the question is that easy. Of course we all surely want more people to be treated, and if alterations to the skill mix brings that about we should welcome the change.

If the patients are fully informed and consulted on the changes in practice and are willing to receive treatment from the private company, so be it. My friends had not thought that the patients could be consulted, but agreed with me that they should be. Can it be right to profit from people who are ill? Because the company that won the contract will not be able to stay in business unless it makes a profit, I wonder what the users of the dialysis think of companies making profit out of their misfortune? Are the patients just grateful to be receiving treatment, or have they never been asked what they feel about anything to do with their health before, and therefore feel that they have no right to comment now? What I mean by empowerment is encouraging patients to have a say in their treatment and how it is delivered. This can be achieved by encouraging patient groups to come and meet nursing staff, become involved in support groups and develop patient forums at local or national level, in order to be able to ask direct questions concerning how they feel about the standard of care they are receiving.

Surely we should be able to ask users what they need and expect from their nurses. Much is said and written about ADVOCACY and in particular the role of the nurse as the patients' advocate. Recent examples of nurses speaking out for patients' rights, or commenting on worrying standards of pratice, have been met with a hostile response from management. The case of Mr Graham Pink comes to mind as a good example of what can happen to those who take on the role of the advocate. He was drawing attention to severe staff shortage on his acute care of the elderly ward. Nurses have been affected by his case, and the climate within the present health service is creating an atmosphere of 'accepting the system as it is because it could be your job next'. The RCN has been operating a confidential 'whistleblowing' service for nurses, which is very much needed. It is, however, so depressing that in a country that prides itself on its democracy, having a large number of its citizens as practising professionals with an accompanying body of knowledge and skills, attending conferences and study days, and involved in continuing education, these same people are still to a very large degree unable to stand up and say locally, or nationally, that they are very concerned about standards of practice. In other words, we are not practising as the patients' advocates and we should not fool ourselves and toss the word around as if it were an accepted part of our professional life.

Karen Jennings (1991) also raises some challenging issues. She discusses the enormous responsibilities of the average registered nurse: '. . . the pressing demands of the nurse will dilute and detract from the role of the advocate. In fact, the term advocacy is in danger of becoming a buzz-word, a fashionable trend, which will only serve to bring into question our professional integrity. I say this because, if nurses are advocates, then we have clearly failed in that role . . . The evidence for that failure abounds on city pavements throughout the country. Over the last ten years, large numbers of patients have been discharged from psychiatric hospitals to sub-standard accommodation and many have drifted into homelessness and despair as a result. It was nurses who were involved in the process of discharge.' She goes on to suggest that 'Patient advocacy is essential, but is it essential that nurses do it? Perhaps as a profession we should wake up to the conflicts within our roles as nurses and within the system and foster an independent advocacy service that will be able to represent the patients interests objectively.'

Mental health has always been grossly underfunded and without a clear strategy for the development of an integrated service that is needs led. Nurses who work in the mental health field have also been made to feel that their contribution to health care is of a different status to general, more appealing medicine and nursing. In many instances they attempt to repair the damage inflicted on people because of unemployment, poverty, and homelessness. How can nurses respect and empower patients if they do not feel valued and empowered themselves? An excellent document on *Guidelines for Empowering Users of Mental Health Services* was jointly sponsored by COHSE and MIND. The document has an interesting approach to real partnership in care.

UNEMPLOYMENT OF NURSES

Question: 'So what do you want to be when you leave nursing school?'
Answer: 'A Staff Nurse in my training hospital please.'
Response: 'Sorry nurse, there is no work for you today, despite the fact that at least £36,000 has been spent on your last three year's of training.'

Four years ago there was such a serious shortage of nurses that the Department of Health launched a £4.5 million recruitment campaign on television, costing £20,000 for every student who enrolled for training. A vast majority of applications for NHS Trust status proclaimed that 'staff are our most valuable resource'. It is little wonder that thousands of nurses throughout the country find that this statement is difficult to accept.

The Royal College of Nursing has said that millions of pounds has been wasted training nurses who now have no prospect of work. Colleges of Nursing have recruited too many students in the absence of central guidance in the Government's NHS reforms and the new-style, market-led health service where self governing Trusts decide staff levels. Consultant health cuts are costing nursing jobs in the NHS. Nearly 8,500 nursing jobs have disappeared since the introduction of the NHS reforms, as new Government figures show. The Government has refused to release a total redundancy figure or to break the information down into staff grades. Region-by-region breakdown of staff shows that between 1989 and 1991 – the most critical period of the Government's health reforms and the internal market – the number of whole-time equivalents in nursing and midwifery fell by 8,420. The number of managers and office staff went up by 17,110 (Milburn, 1991). The Department of Health stated that the decrease in the number of nurses could be explained by senior nurses moving to the managerial pay spine. This was strongly disputed by Christine Hancock, RCN General Secretary. The figures call fundamentally into question the NHS reforms' ability to bring services closer to the patient. Increasingly the very important Trusts, which are so alive to the need to employ rising numbers of senior managers, seem to believe both that there is no need for nurses more senior than the ward sister, and that they can make do with fewer qualified clinical staff, although nurses are of proven benefit to patient care and managers are not. Karen Jennings, COHSE Professional Officer, agreed 'The department explanation cannot possibly hold water. COHSE is backing a call made by Alan Milburn MO, for the National Audit Office, to examine the efficiency and effectiveness of the new managers.'

Staffing changes in NHS regions 1989–1991

	Managers	Admin/clerical	Nursing/midwifery
Northern	+600	+430	−530
Yorkshire	+610	+590	−660
Trent	+510	+800	−150
East Anglia	+310	+560	−420
North West Thames	+590	+400	−330
North East Thames	+770	+900	−140
South East Thames	+690	+1040	−1070

South West Thames	+390	+300	−1350
Wessex	+440	+650	+210
Oxford	+320	+70	−130
South Western	+390	+1080	−130
West Midlands	+910	+940	−830
Mersey	+440	+370	−1860
North Western	+640	+1370	−1030
Total	+7610	+9500	−8420

(Carlisle, 1993)

Raising the Political Profile of Nursing

Nursing is not only influenced by politics, it can and does influence politics itself. Some nurses have become very politically involved. They have stood as candidates for political parties at both local and national level. Some of these nurses have been successful at local level and are very involved in local government politics. At national level they have yet to be successful. They must all be congratulated, for their courage and commitment and for behaving in a truly accountable and professional manner. When a parliamentary candidate myself, I was asked at a public meeting why I wanted to change my job, from one as a nurse, which has high public respect and ethical credibility, to that of an MP, which has little or no public respect and practises questionable ethics. My answer was on the lines of change. Many politicians are very credible, honest and have a strong desire to bring about a high quality of life and justice for the people that they represent. Nursing enables us to demonstrate many of the skills a 'good' politician should have. These include being a good communicator, having problem-solving ability, being a team player, encouraging independence, being capable of making difficult decisions, exercising high standards of practice, respecting confidentiality and treating all people equally. Nurses bring much needed credibility to politics, so why are political nurses still viewed with much suspicion? One could say that ethics is about feeling comfortable with what is happening around you. How many nurses can say that?

I want to examine next the nurses' personal and professional responsibility to speak out. Society generally does not trust anyone much who challenges the *status quo*, and nursing is exceptionally hostile to such people. Ironically, nurses who kick up a fuss, lose their temper, or fight for patients' rights overtly, are often labelled deviant, stupid, politically extreme or unprofessional. Only nursing could find itself equating professionalism with acquiesence, subservience, silence, and obedience (*see* Jolley and Brykczynska, 1993). 'Members of other professions would take great pride in a collective battle in which individual differences were subsumed into a common interest' (Clay, 1987).

I have never made any secret about being political, or encouraging nurses to be very aware of political influences within their private and working life. I do not want to turn the clinical domain into a public political battleground. Having political banners at the bedside is not what being politically aware is all about. But as nurses we do see the daily effect that politics has on people. We know that huge inequalities in health and health care exist. The recent Government paper *The Health of the Nation* ignores the fact that the link between poverty, unemployment, housing and other quality of life issues have on the health of the nation (Department of Health, 1992).

As has been stated above, we live and work in rapidly changing times. The whole nursing profession is moving forward in terms of standards within a new educational framework. This is being encouraged by nursing leaders in clinical practice and education. But nurses at the bedside are being constrained in developing the new knowledge and skills necessary by their employing organizations, other professionals, and even by their own colleagues. This may restrict their freedom to question and challenge. However the new UKCC learning outcomes for all Project 2000 courses are statutory, for example, the recognition of common factors which contribute adversely to physical, mental and social well-being of patients and clients (United Kingdom Central Council for Nursing, 1989).

Nurse educationalists have the responsibility of providing leadership to students. All nurses need to stand together to implement change. Together we truly would be a force for change, united we are all strong — divided we will all fall.

CONCLUSION

A couple of weeks after the 1992 General Election I set off to watch my local football team play. As I approached the ground I felt for the loose change in my pocket that I always carry with me, to buy a match programme, and give the change to the regular charities and voluntary groups that are usually at the entrance to the ground collecting for their local cause. As I got nearer I could see that the collectors this week were nurses. They were in uniform complete with caps. It was raining, and they were holding buckets, rattling the coins and asking people to support their local hospital.

I was embarrassed, angry and almost close to tears as I stood back and watched ordinary working people — young and old — dropping coins into their buckets. I looked at the nurses' faces, they looked, understandably, fed up and were getting very wet. I pulled myself together and went over to chat. I asked them what, in particular, they were collecting for. They replied that they were under the impression that it was for new surgical equipment. They said that they felt embarrassed collecting in this way but there was nothing else they could do as the equipment was needed. I sat through the football game oblivious to the play until the end, when we knew that our team would soon be playing in the First Division next season. It was then that I remembered that the Government had announced a 'hospital league table' which would be published and presumably improve competition. Well, my football team would never have reached Division One if the staff and fans of the club had been forced to stand outside the ground every week collecting money for equipment, training, or even players!

The staff at my local hospital are very well able to be in Division One — some should be in the Premier League! The hospital building on the other hand should be demolished and rebuilt, staff and patients have a very poor environment in which to practise and stay, unlike the carefully nurtured pitch that the 'lads' play on. I believe the referee should show the red card to the Health Minister, and the rest of the team and send them off for committing a most serious professional foul. Yes, I am biased. Locally, I can be heard shouting 'come on, you Reds'. Nationally, I shout the same – I am interested in the game, in fact, more than interested. I want to play for the First Team. There are others out there who could also play. Some will need some extra coaching, some are injured but will soon be 'fit' to play. The 'game' of politics most definitely needs new players, the fans deserve better. The new players may wear different coloured strips and supporters will choose which team to support. All we need now is for nursing and its organizations to put forward the transfer fee . . .

REFERENCES

Bagust, A. and Oakley, J. (1992) *Ward Nursing Quality and Grade-Mix Report of Paired Ward Experiments Undertaken in the North Western Region.* Final Report. North Western RHA, Manchester.

Bevan, A. (1952) *In Place of Fear.* Heinemann, London.

Bevan, S. and Stock, J. (1991) *Choosing and Approach to Reprofiling and Skill Mix.* Institute of Manpower Studies, Brighton.

Buchan, J. and Ball, J. (1991) *Caring Costs.* Institute of Manpower Studies, Brighton.

Carlisle, D. (1993) Clinical jobs fall while the number of managers rises. *Nursing Times,* 89(2), 6.

Carr-Hill, R., Dixon, P., Gibbs, I., Griffiths, M., Higgins, M., McCaughan, D. and Wright, K. (1992) *Skill Mix and the Effectiveness of Nursing Care.* Centre for Health, University of York, York.

Clay, T. (1987) *Nurses: Power and Politics.* Heinemann, London.

Department of Health (1991) *The Patient's Charter.* HMSO, London.

Department of Health (1992) *The Health of the Nation.* HMSO, London.

Department of Health and Social Security (1986) *Mix and Match: a Review of Nursing Skill Mix.* (DHSS, London). (Chairman P. Wright-Warren).

Dyson, R. (1991) *Changing Labour Utilisation in NHS Trusts: the Reprofiling Paper.* University of Keele, Centre for Health Planning and Management, Keele.

Friend, B. (1991) The storyteller. *Nursing Times,* 887(38), 16.

Gibbs, I., McCaughan, D. and Griffiths, M. (1990) *Skill Mix in Nursing: a Selective Review of the Literature.* Centre for Health Economics, University of York, York.

Jennings, K. (1991) Speaking up for patients. *COHSE Journal,* 3(5), 12–3.

Kelly, T.A. and O'Leary, M. (1992) *Nursing Skill Mix in the District Nursing Service.* HMSO, London.

National Union of Public Employees (1993) *Skill Mix and Reprofiling in the Health Service: NUPE Guidelines*. NUPE, London.
Seymour, J. (1992) Pick and mix. *Nursing Times*, 88(33), 19.

7.

CARE IN THE YEAR 2000

Someone once said that prophecy is very difficult, particularly with regard to the future. Nevertheless, two years ago, on the occasion the Royal College of Nursing's 75th anniversary, I outlined a vision of the future for patient care and the challenges in store for nurses. In a special publication (Hancock, 1991) I wrote that the patient of the future could be sitting at a computer screen in her or his own home keying in codes to 'beam up' a nurse for advice. This may seem a far-fetched vision of the future of health care. But in fact it is a scenario that rests on some basic assumptions and predictions about the future of care that many nurses are working towards now.

The idea of the modern patient assumes that, in future, we will be a healthier and more equal society. Many more people will have access to health care and health education – a vision also shared by the World Health Organization when it outlined its *Health for All by the Year 2000* targets (WHO, 1981), some 15 years ago.

Those people will be generally more choosy, demanding and knowledgable about their health, and nurses will have a real health promotion role in the health service. Health care will be firmly focused in the community – on people's homes, in schools, and in workplaces.

Nurses are well placed to meet the wider health needs of the population. For too long, and despite all the attention now being paid to prevention and health promotion, our health services have primarily been sickness services. Most resources have been devoted to last-minute repairing of problems which could have been prevented or treated earlier.

A key performance indicator of success in most countries is the increase in the number of people who are being treated in hospitals, even though hospital treatments are marginal to the health of the population.

Meanwhile, health care is still very much defined as medical care. For nurses, such a definition does not always recognize the contribution that they make to patient well-being. Yet today, and as we head for the next century, the fact remains that we are more likely to suffer from mental illness than from physical. The biggest killers are cardiovascular incidents followed by cancers and road accidents. But with the prevalence of HIV and AIDS, and widespread poverty and home-lessness, infectious diseases are once again threatening the health of large sections of the population.

Medical intervention, that is, short-term life-saving intervention – will always be necessary. But it is less effective in the control, management and treatment of infection. Health education about lifestyle, diet and environment is a more effective and considerably cheaper way to control disease, including heart disease, and to promote the long-term health of the nation.

For those whose lives are saved or who benefit from medical intervention, the period of adjustment to a new condition, to a permanently altered state of mind or body, or intensive care in hospital, requires nursing care and management.

And increasingly, if patients do need hospital care as opposed to day care to receive medical treatment, it will be precisely because they need nursing care. That is, they will require skilled observation and help to perform the essential activities of breathing, eating and moving around.

Meanwhile, greater 'consumerism' has also had an impact on health care, leading to the de-medicalization of certain services. For instance, midwifery-led services for women are back and fully supported by the recent Government report on maternity care (The House of Commons Health Committee, 1992).

The greater use of the Domino (DOMiciliary IN–Out) system in midwifery places the emphasis on individualized community care. Parents now have greater access to children in hospital. In both cases pressure from consumers has sought to make health care professionals 'partners in care'.

In this way, nursing is empowering consumers, enabling them to make healthy choices about the way they live their lives. In some countries this partnership has been developed to the benefit of nurses and clients alike. In New Zealand, midwives in particular have been able to call on patients for support, offering them associate membership of their professional association and regularly sending them information on changes in practice and the health service. In this way, a health partnership between nurse and patient has been established, and all nurses enjoy very high levels of public support.

Here in the UK a number of branches of nursing have forged links with patient self-help groups. Others have mobilized the public to campaign with them. For example, in the West of England, when a new child health strategy proposed cuts in the school nursing service, school nurses wrote not only to GPs outlining the implications of the cuts, but distributed letters to parents through teachers. So far, they have received strong support. Consequently, nursing's valuable and unique contribution to people's health is being reflected in Government health strategies and recognised in a growing number of research studies. Also, nursing itself is creating new models within which independent practitioners are professional, intelligent members of the health care team with an individual and crucial contribution to make to that team.

In the foreseeable future, as the numbers and dependency levels of priority groups in the community increase, so demand for the services of a wide range of community nurses will increase. Well-documented demographic data shows a steep growth in the numbers of very old frail people over 85 years who will require more care. At the other end of the spectrum, the increase in the number of children under five over the next three years alone will require an extra 2.5 % growth in nursing numbers.

As traditional in-patient care becomes the exception rather than the rule, higher levels of day surgery – intensive, high-dependency work – will require increased levels of staffing in hospitals and effective community support. But there are serious challenges to be overcome if our health services are to respond to these changes and really to focus on providing the health care that people want and need; and meeting these challenges depends on the wider recognition of the contribution of nursing to the health of the nation.

We live in an era of cost constraint and work within a health care system in which, like the commercial sector, competition has heightened awareness of costs for purchasers and providers alike. Over the last two years, increasing numbers of patients have been treated with fewer qualified nurses. Many are concerned that such staffing changes in hospitals are merely a reaction to short-term funding considerations rather than based on a longer-term analysis of care and nursing needs.

The NHS has lacked a strategy for staffing the health service, lurching regularly from shortage to glut depending on prevailing economic circumstances. In a recession nurses may be less mobile and less able to find work outside the NHS, while in periods of greater prosperity, the nurse may vote with her feet.

A national strategy which looks in a focused and imaginative way at the skill-base needed for tomorrow's health service, and a strategy for retaining qualified nurses, are both urgently required as we approach the year 2000.

Qualified nurses are adaptable, flexible and skilled practitioners. They are able to update their skills or learn new ones at short notice. A health service seeking cost effective, high-quality care must keep those skills and enable nurses to acquire new ones. Nevertheless, as the largest group of staff in the National Health Service, consuming some 3% of public expenditure, nurses accept that in a context of financial constraint it is legitimate to ask them to demonstrate their value. And they are doing so.

Now, there is an expanding body of evidence that proves an undeniable link between the number of qualified nurses employed and the quality of care received by patients. *Caring Costs* (Buchan and Ball, 1991) was the first British review of US and UK research studies to show the benefits of employing qualified nurses. Commissioned by the Royal College of Nursing, an Institute of Manpower Studies research team identified a broad group of studies which consider the relationship between cost and quality, and the cost effectiveness of clinical interventions by specialist nurses. It also considers the cost effectiveness of non-clinical nurse interventions where qualified nurses have rationalized the use of resources through more efficient stock-taking and the redesign of patient documentation.

A number of independent studies have since examined the relationship between the employment of qualified nurses and quality care. A York University report, *Ward Nursing Quality and Grade Mix* (Bagust et al, 1992) indicated that high standards of care depend on using qualified nurses. In the first phase of the two-year study, the authors worked with nurses to produce a Quality Pointer Tool to assess what happens on a ward when the level of care falls. The report concludes that in grade-mix exercises that are purely cost driven, cash savings must be paid for with poorer quality.

A report commissioned by the Department of Health and undertaken by York University Centre for Health Economics (Carr-Hill et al, 1992) concludes that investment in obtaining qualified staff, providing post qualification training and developing an effective method of organizing care, pays dividends in the delivery of a high standard of patient care.

An American study commissioned by the US Department of Health and Human Services (Robinson and Luft, 1987) concludes: 'Although nurse staffing levels are highly visible items on hospital balance sheets, they are also highly visible indices of hospital quality from the perspectives of patients, physicians and insurance plans. Given the important role that nurse staffing and skill mix play in competition among hospitals, managers must resist the short-term temptation to cut personnel costs to the point where long-term losses in market share results'

A number of the studies contained in *Caring Costs* look at ways of calculating nurse productivity. One study by Helt and Jelinek (1988) showed that, although a higher proportion of registered nurses led to an increase in labour costs, the subsequent increase in productivity meant an overall cost saving through a reduction in nursing hours.

In addition, the NHS Management Executive's new methodology for comparing performance – the *Labour Productivity Index* (1992) – has been piloted in a number of NHS sites. It compares activity levels with staff costs and output. Reports from these sites state: 'Higher rates of pay do not necessarily mean higher labour costs. Higher productivity meant lower Unit Labour Costs and higher numbers of qualified staff employed resulted in lower Unit Labour Costs'.

Caring Costs also highlights a number of studies and reviews that show the cost-effectiveness of nursing skills where they are substituted for other professional skills. One review of the cost-effectiveness of nurses includes a study comparing physicians and nurse practitioners in the United States (Ramsay 1986). It indicates that nurse practitioners are better able to control their patients' obesity and hypertension. Furthermore, patients respond better to follow-up treatment.

Another study highlights the cost effectiveness of midwives. Minor in his study of 1989, showed the average cost of a midwife's services to be $994 compared with a physician's fee of $1,492.

The RCN recently commissioned an independent research paper, which highlights the significant cost savings that could result from employing qualified nurses and nurse practitioners in general practice (Marsh 1991). Some GPs have argued that, with appropriately qualified nurses, a GP could manage a list of 4,000 people instead of the present UK average of 1,870.

Discussion of cost benefits does not apply to staffing only, but to care settings, for example, the cost benefits of home care as an alternative to hospital. Here in the UK, 'Hospitals at Home', which deliver high level intensive nursing in the home for people who would otherwise have to occupy an expensive hospital bed have been evaluated. Evaluation of a scheme that has been operating in Peterborough since 1978 (Marks, 1991) shows more rapid rates of rehabilitation than those patients who have conventional hospital post-operative care. Another Hospital at Home, established in Pembroke in 1991, showed a saving for the orthopaedic unit of about five days per patient. For elderly patients with a fractured neck of the femur, a total bed-saving of 38 days was recorded.

Research on community care provision for elderly people published by the RCN's Daphne Heald Research Unit shows that elderly people value the work of community nurses very highly and that these nurses play a key role in reducing unnecessary drug consumption amongst older people (Wade 1993).

In future, working with GPs and other health care professionals in primary health care teams, nurses could realistically completely restructure the concept of hospital care, creating a service that begins and ends in the community. But if we are to realize the potential of primary health care we need to ensure the development of a real partnership between GP and nurse – a partnership in which team members work together on an equal footing, recognizing the individual skills and roles of their colleagues. In this way they could ensure that they target and meet the needs of the whole community.

Alongside the statistics on cost effectiveness, the Royal College of Nursing published the *Value of Nursing* (1992) report, which provides a qualitative record of the real-life experiences of nurses whose care has dramatically improved the quality of lives of their patients, and in many cases, their lives.

In many ways, this type of qualitative work is as essential as the quantitative data. It identifies the invisible aspects of nursing care which nevertheless make such an important contribution to the recovery and future well-being of patients. Yet it is because of the invisible nature of so much nursing practice – the fact that good nursing is often about making people feel that they are not being nursed at all – that nursing has traditionally been labelled as a 'low-tech' occupation.

At the same time, the highly technological and heroic treatment so often associated with medicine and other professions allied to medicine has afforded them a much higher status within the health care team.

Winning the arguments on quality and cost effectiveness are certainly essential in raising the status of nursing and ensuring that in future it is recognized as an important professional discipline in its own right. But achieving this professional status also means overcoming the low social status that is still associated with it. This status is traditionally reflected by low pay, poor conditions and occupational powerlessness. Many analysts have highlighted the fact that the accepted female and subservient nature of nursing undermines efforts to establish professional status.

As Moya Jolley highlights in Chapter 5, the concepts of the nurse as a woman and the woman or mother as a nurse have become integrated. They form an image of nursing that militates against its professionalism. As nursing sets its course for the next century, the fact remains that it is carrying a lot of excess baggage from the past. As Jolley points out, passive, feminine images of nursing have been distorted and perpetuated through the media.

Some unpublished RCN research looked at the attitudes of decision makers in broadcasting towards nurses and nursing. The people questioned were programme makers, scriptwriters and producers of news and current affairs programmes, documentaries, dramas and drama series. The survey confirmed previous evidence that nurses are seen as victims. They are useful for crisis stories. But they were not seen as suitable members of expert panels. So it is no wonder we don't often see a nurse explaining to the public the advantages of new technologies or treatment, or even commenting on health issues and health promotion.

Interestingly, and perhaps surprisingly, in the field of television drama, it seems that things are beginning to change. In the UK's top soap, *Coronation Street*, there is currently a long-running and very positive story line about a mature nursing student. Although the character is a man, when this story line began, colleges of nursing all over the UK received a large number of enquiries from men and women who had identified a positive role model.

And in the UK's most successful hospital drama series, *Casualty*, it is not unusual to see a nurse correctly challenging a doctor's diagnosis.

Back in reality, growing confidence about the value of nursing care has enabled nurses to make important inroads in establishing themselves professionally as the cornerstone of health care by the year 2000.

A workforce that is valued and valuable is any organization's greatest asset. Low salaries, low morale and poor working conditions have always militated against quality and professionalism – in all sectors. Nurses pay in the UK fell in real value during the early 1980s and nurses lobbied hard to secure new procedures for determining pay. The Pay Review Body established in 1983 led to an increase in nursing salaries in real terms, and pay has risen by 28 per cent since 1984. In 1988, a graded pay structure was introduced to reward nurses for their skills and level of responsibility. Despite its clumsy implementation, the long-term benefits of this type of structure are obvious.

FURTHER DEVELOPMENTS

Project 2000 was the result of many years of dissatisfaction with traditional methods of training nurses. The curriculum supports the development of skilled, competent, self-motivated practitioners with a focus on health promotion and an understanding of the future demands of health care.

Alan Myles' assessment of the 'vintage practitioner' in chapter 2 takes an optimistic but realistic look at the future of nurse education. While traditional training has restricted the ability of the hospital nurse to work in the community, Project 2000 paves the way for a more flexible practitioner.

Given that most of the workforce for the 1990s and the beginning of the next century are already in jobs, post-registration education and practice will also be essential in realizing their full potential.

The wider implementation of the named nurse initiative as part of the Patients' Charter was an important affirmation by the Government of the value of nursing. It represents essential recognition of the benefits to patients of knowing that a qualified nurse is responsible for their care, from admission, before, and throughout the period of care to discharge and beyond.

Meanwhile, increasing numbers of nurses are participating in quality assurance initiatives and standard setting. In 1985 the Royal College of Nursing established the Dynamic Quality Improvement Programme to enable nurses and other health care professionals to set and develop their own standards.

The quality framework is implemented through the Dynamic Standard Setting System (RCN, 1990), through which nurses, with their colleagues, managers and educators, actually define acceptable standards of care across the spectrum of nursing specialities.

Despite the delay in its implementation, nurse prescribing legislation is already on the statute book. In fact, many community nurses already play an active role in prescribing, either by protocol, through recommendations to the GP, or by recommending over-the-counter products directly to clients. As nursing practice becomes increasingly advanced and more diverse, nurses will inevitably be able to enhance the care they give, prescribing in more and more areas of health care. Indeed, the extension and development of nursing practice based on research and innovation is another example of the changing face of nursing in response to the health care challenges of the 1990s.

One of the earliest attempts to develop nursing practice by putting research findings into practice was the 1986 study into the effects of caring for elderly people in a therapeutic nursing unit in at Burford in Oxfordshire (Pearson, 1987). Nurses in the unit were responsible for planning and providing intensive, patient-centered, holistic care. Patients discharged from the unit were less dependent than other patients and experienced higher standards of care during their treatment. On average, length of stay was shorter in the treatment unit and some 73% of patients in the nursing unit had no complaints at all about their care, compared with 41 % in the control unit. In addition, there was evidence that on average, costs per day in the nursing unit were significantly lower.

Now, teams of nurses throughout the country are receiving money from the King's Fund to become Nursing Development Units (NDUs), enabling them to extend existing nursing practice and develop new and effective models of care.

The first community NDU to be funded by the King's Fund was established at Strelley Health Centre outside Nottingham. The team of health visitors covers five estates where social disadvantage and unemployment are much higher than the national average. The area has the highest death and discharge rates in the county for paediatrics and general surgery as well as above average numbers of low-weight births, coronary heart disease and strokes.

The health visitors at Strelley have provided support networks to improve the health of local women and to reduce child accident rates. .

The team is able to gather important information, such as a survey of local nurseries, which revealed that 500 children in the area were on waiting lists for nursery places. And partnerships have been established with colleagues in housing, social and environmental services.

The work of the Strelley NDU demonstrates how high-quality, cost-effective preventative health care can be provided in the community. The team is effectively profiling the community using a genuine public health approach to collecting epidemiological data. In future, nurses will be invaluable in collecting this type of data and, together with GPs, will be able to plan the implementation of strategies for health promotion and health gain throughout the community.

Nursing practice is also developing in new directions in the hospital setting. With the reduction of junior doctor hours and the publication of the UKCC's *Scope of Professional Practice* (1992), the overlap between the roles of doctors and nurses has been widely debated. One area where this relationship has quickly taken on new dimensions is cardiac surgery. The Royal College of Surgeons recently produced a report on the use of surgeons' assistants in certain routine procedures (Holmes, 1994).

Some surgeons have applauded the scheme as an effective way of reducing junior doctor hours and improving standards of care. The use of nurses as surgeons' assistants does not offer a solution to the question of junior doctor hours, and they are certainly not a cheap option. Rather, this is and must be seen as one of many developments in advanced nursing practice. In this area as in many others, the holistic approach of nursing to the care of patients is invaluable.

Now almost every unit can provide examples of nurses who are undertaking work that was traditionally part of the medical domain. For example, nurses are running their own out-patient clinics, have access to nursing beds and are substituting for doctors by agreement in a whole range of activities from intravenous therapy to verification of death. Midwifery-led services for women are back and fully supported by the recent Government report on maternity care.

A number of studies show that given the choice, patients often prefer to see a nurse before or instead of a doctor. Consequently, there is a growing interest in the potential for developing nurse practitioners in hospitals and the community.

Health Authorities such as South East Thames Regional Health Authority have ackowledged that nurses working at nurse practitioner level can work effectively in high street chemists as well as out in the community with people who are not registered with a general practitioner, including groups of homeless people, for example.

In a number of cities nurse practitioners are actually working with homeless people. Many of their clients have chronic alcohol-related problems and a history of mental illness. Most have no other access to health care. Increasingly, nurse practitioners will be a valuable extra resource for the development of new areas of care.

The expanding role of the nurse practitioner has led a number of nurses and GPs to explore the desirability of forming a partnership in which the nurse practitioner literally becomes a partner with a financial interest in the practice. Whether or not this will actually happen in the UK either before or after the year 2000, I believe that at the very least, nurse practitioners should seek parity with their GPs. They need to work together on an equal footing, recognizing the individual skills and respecting the different educational and practice traditions of their colleagues.

In a growing number of hospitals, the role and practice of nursing has been dramatically affected most recently by the reorganization of care using the patient-focused hospital initiative. This concept, first devised in the United States, has serious implications for the nursing workforce as we approach the year 2000.

Health care staff in this country have expressed concern about the way it has been interpreted in the UK. Many believe that it has been seen by many health service managers purely as a way of saving money in the short term, and that patients' needs are being broken down into a series of tasks to be carried out by a member of a team of all-purpose personnel.

Strangely, health service managers in this country, who in recent years seem to have had an insatiable appetite for all things Stateside, seem to be less interested in American nursing experience. Evidence from the most successful patient-focused units in the United States reveals the pivotal role of nursing staff in making the initiative work.

In the most progressive units in the United States, on the whole, team leaders and unit managers are nurses.

A study of the care teams at Lakeland Medical Centre in the United States reveals that each team contains nurses, therapists, student nurses and health care assistants working in partnership.

Multi-skilling is explained as giving out the dinners and making beds as well as undertaking ECGs and helping with X-rays. So the cost savings achieved from patient focus do not come from the dilution of the care teams' skill mix or through employing less qualified care staff.

When the Chief Nurse Executive at Lakeland, Phyllis Watson, was interviewed about the initiative, she stressed that nursing roles were not blurred or disaggregated in cross-trained teams, but rather enhanced as the needs of patients were matched with the skills of staff when building a care team. She said: 'We only cross-train skills and not professional decision making. We don't believe that we can cross-train the knowledge and experience that is essential to make adequate decisions. Furthermore, we only cross-train a skill if we identify that there is adequate volume of that skill to maintain competency over a period of time. If the volume is inadequate, we provide focused staff to perform this skill and do not cross-train it. We never cross-train skills that require previously established professional requirements.'

Clearly, the value of the care team lies not in creating a group of generic health care workers with interchangeable skills, but in reflecting the different individual professional strengths that are derived from different educational and practice traditions.

Consequently, evaluation by Brider (1992) in the *American Journal of Nursing* reveals that although there are some concerns about the initiative, in a number of units the time that staff have available for patients has increased, length of stay has shortened and admission and turnaround for routine tests has speeded up significantly. If the motivation for implementing patient focus is the need to improve quality and provide cost effective care, rather than short-term cost savings, hospitals in this country will need to understand that nurse staffing and skill levels will increasingly mean the difference between success and failure.

So, where is nursing headed as we approach 2000? If initiatives like 'patient focus' have the wrong focus and short-term cost considerations are central to decisions on staff and resource allocation, the deskilling of nursing work could have disastrous effects on patient care. And without some form of strategic planning for the nursing workforce, the skills and experience of thousands of nurses could be lost to the NHS at a time when they are needed more than ever.

Meeting health needs in the year 2000, the ability to assess care needs, to prescribe treatment and constantly to update skills as technology demands, requires the competence and experience of a qualified nurse. Government health policy has already stated the need for more nursing resources in the future in the community. The ability of the NHS to provide high-quality, cost-effective care in the next century depends on it.

Nursing, and perhaps only nursing, has the ability to deliver a reforming health agenda that is flexible and responsive to the patient, which delivers care in the most appropriate setting, which empowers patients to take charge of their own health and that is cost effective. As we move towards the next century, we will find that nursing's time has come.

REFERENCES

Bagust, A., Oakley, J. and Slack, R. (1992) *Ward Nursing Quality and Grade Mix.* North Western Regional Health Authority, Manchester.

Brider, P. (1992) The move to patient focused care. *American Journal of Nursing,* 92(9), 26–33.

Buchan, J. and Ball, J. (1991) *Caring Costs: Nursing Costs and Benefits.* Institute of Manpower Studies, Brighton.

Carr-Hill, R., Dixon, P., Gibbs, I., Griffiths, M., Higgins, M., McCaughan, D. and Wright, K. (1992) *Skill Mix and the Effectiveness of Nursing Care.* Centre for Health Economics, University of York, York.

Hancock, C. (1991) Looking to a future role. In *Royal College of Nursing: Seventy Five Years Strong,* pp.2–3. RCN, London.

Helt, E.H. and Jelinek, R.C. (1988) In the wake of cost cutting, nursing producitivity and quality improve. *Nursing Management,* 19(6), 36–48.

Holmes, S. (1994) Development of the cardiac surgeon's assistant. *British Journal of Nursing,* 3(5),

House of Commons. Health Committee (1992) Maternity Services. Volume 1: Report. HMSO, London. (Chairman N. Winterton).

Marks, L. (1991) *Home and Hospital Care: Re-drawing the Boundaries.* Kings Fund Institute, London.

Minor, A.F. (1989) *The Cost of Maternity Care and Childbirth in the United States.* Health Insurance Association of America, Washington.

Pearson, A. (Ed.) (1987) *Primary Nursing: Nursing in the Burford and Oxford Nursing Development Unit.* Croom Helm, London.

Marsh, G. (1991) Future of general practice. Caring for larger lists. *British Medical Journal,* 303, 1312–6.

Ramsay, J.A. (1986) Physicians and nurse practitioners: do they provide equivalent healthcare? *American Journal of Public Health,* 72, 55–6.

Robinson, J.C. and Luft, H.S. (1987) Competition and the Cost of Hospital Care. *Journal of the American Hospital Association,* 257, 3241–5.

Royal College of Nursing (1990). *Quality Patient Care: The Dynamic Standard Setting System.* RCN, London.

Royal College of Nursing (1992). *The Value of Nursing.* RCN, London.

Tomlinson, B. (1992). Report of the Inquiry into London's Health Serrvice, Medical Education and Research. HMSO, London.

United Kingdom Central Council for Nursing, Midwifery and Health Visiting (1992) *The Scope of Professional Practice: a UKCC Position Statement*. UKCC, London.

Wade, B. (1993) *The Chaing Face of Community Care for Older People: Year 1, Setting the Scene*. Daphne Heald Research Unit, Royal College of Nursing, London.

World Health Organization (1981) *Health for All by the Year 2000*. WHO, Geneva.

INDEX